I0467929

YOUR ER SURVIVAL GUIDE

Kathleen A. Handal, MD

Published by DocHandal, LLC

ISBN 13 - 9781500506483

DocHandal, LLC publishes first aid, health and safety materials in a variety of electronic formats. Discounts for bulk orders and customized editions may be available from the publisher.

DISCLAIMER: This is a guide to assist when considering medical assistance for an emergency. The author does not represent that every acceptable facet of seeking emergency medical care is contained herein or those abnormal or unusual circumstances may not warrant or require additional activities. This material is not designed to take the place of a visit to a medical care facility or evaluation by a physician. Doc Handal recommends that you read this long before you have to seek medical care in an ER.

The information within this guide is a compilation of general ER operational aspects and information reflecting the current features, knowledge and accepted emergency medicine practice in the United States at the time this guide was published. The reader is urged to learn about their local area's emergency medical resources.

ABOUT THE AUTHOR

Kathleen Handal, MD is a nationally and internationally known emergency medicine "Doc". She authored "The American Red Cross First Aid & Safety Handbook" which was written for consumers.

Doc believes physicians have a responsibility to teach and share medical common sense. Up to recently her website, www.Dochandal.com and podcast channel – Doc Handal Speaks! Listen Up – serve as bases for her many consumer education endeavors. A frequent host and co-host on talk-radio health shows, she has also appeared on CNN and the Today Show. Her "Medical Emergencies in the Workplace" video won a bronze medal in the International Cindy Competition and was a Telly Award finalist. She has co-authored a series of medical textbooks.

As part of her dedication to public education, she wrote, directed and produced "Trauma Run", a nationally distributed video for grades 2-6. The video, produced in Spanish and English, teaches children how to respond to a medical emergency when no adults are available.

Her latest endeavor is the launch of Doc Handal Guides, an affordable series of medical books on topics written for consumers. The first book in the series focuses on her emergency medicine expertise. "Doc's First Aid Guide" (English, Spanish and French) outlines the steps a person should take in a variety of emergency situations. All Doc Handal's Guides are available as E-versions and print.

In this " Your ER Survival Guide" she gives valuable insight into the goings-on in an emergency room (ER), so you'll know how to get the best care possible. It's like having Doc Handal at your side when you need her the most.

Acknowledgments

Many thanks to Brian Coonce, Barbara O'Neill-Maguire, RN, PhD, Maria Allo, MD, FACS, FCCM, Sue Viall, RN-BSN,CMR, John Meser,DO, Howard Fleishon, MD, MMM, FACR and all the ER teams' members who over the years contributed to helping me make a difference.

CONTENTS

INTRODUCTION

Few people get through life without at least one trip to the emergency room (ER), either as a patient or support person for a family member or friend. If you've already experienced your first visit you're probably dreading the idea of ever having to return. "Why is it taking so long?" "What are they doing?" "Why isn't anyone telling me anything?" Remember all those questions that were running through your mind?

Your ER Survival Guide is designed to help calm your fears by addressing these questions and more. After all, who is better equipped to help you than a doctor who worked more than 20 years in the ER? I'm going to give you ten simple steps to follow to get you ready for an ER visit. Then I'll provide you with valuable insight into how an ER operates so you'll know how to get the best care possible. It will be like having Doc Handal at your side when you need her the most.

A trip to the ER is a team effort. I'll introduce you to some of the key players--- doctors, physician assistants, residents, nurses, and technicians--- and explain their roles in your care. They'll be poking, prodding and asking you a lot of questions and possibly running a lot of tests. We'll cover some of the basics and more so you'll have a better understanding of what they're looking for and why.

Remember, too, that you, your family and friends are also part of this team. The care you receive relies heavily on your presentation, your medical history, as well as the current signs and symptoms of your problem, so it's important to be prepared. Taking responsibility for your own health care is key to surviving the ER.

So pay close attention and do what you can now to get ready. No one plans to go to the ER! An ER is a busy place. The doctors and nurses are making decisions in a fast-paced, stressful environment. Mistakes can and do happen. The more you know about what to expect the less likely one of those mistakes will happen to you.

If you came in with a right arm injury and your left arm is placed on the X-ray table, that's an obvious red flag. Ask them why and make sure they've got the correct patient. It's important to ask questions and voice your concerns in a constructive fashion. Screaming and yelling will get you nowhere. If your needs aren't being met, I'll tell you how to move up the chain of command to ensure you're receiving the necessary care. Always take into account that you're not the only one in need of care. Choose your battles wisely!

Once I get you through the ER experience and you're admitted to the hospital, transferred to another hospital, or sent home, what's next? Don't worry; Doc Handal will give you some survival tips for beyond the ER.

As an Emergency Medicine (EM) physician myself, I think you should be aware that Emergency Medicine is a medical specialty, like cardiology. EM doctors (MD and DO) undergo rigorous study and specialty testing throughout their careers. I will be referring to the doctors (same as physicians) who work in the ER as "EM doctors", even though not all the ones you may meet actually have EM board credentials.

Let's get started!

Doc Handal

CHAPTER 1

Be Prepared to Act Quickly and Correctly: Ten Steps

We see two types of patients in the ER. We see patients with sudden onset of an illness or injury, such as victims of a car accident, drowning, stroke or heart attack. Next, we see patients who have had a problem for a while and the signs and symptoms are worsening or not going away, such as redness and swelling in the leg, abdominal pain, and fever. These problems may not be urgent but can have the potential for becoming critical at any time. The appendix that's causing lower quadrant pain and discomfort for hours can burst and become a medical emergency, requiring immediate surgery and antibiotics. Remember, seconds may count and the clock starts ticking long before you get to the ER. Being better prepared you can act quickly and correctly at the first signs of a medical emergency and make all the difference. That's why reading ***Doc's First Aid Guide*** and ***Your ER Survival Guide*** is so important!

Here are ten steps you can take now to get ready for a medical emergency and if necessary a trip to the ER. A detailed explanation of each step will follow.

1. CREATE AN EMERGENCY INFORMATION SHEET (EIS)

2. STOCK YOUR FIRST AID KIT AND YOUR MEDICINE CABINET

3. LEARN FIRST AID AND READ YOUR FIRST AID BOOK

4. MAKE A MEDICAL HISTORY / MEDICATIONS LIST

5. KNOW YOUR INSURANCE COVERAGE

6. GET YOUR LEGAL DOCUMENTS IN ORDER

7. GET TO KNOW YOUR ER

8. PREPARE YOUR CHILDREN FOR THE ER

9. KNOW WHEN TO GO TO THE ER

10. GET READY FOR EMERGENCY MEDICAL SERVICES (EMS)

1. Create an Emergency Info Sheet (EIS)

An EIS is a great timesaver. When minutes count you don't want to be fumbling through the phone book or looking on the web for a phone number. Take the time now to fill in all the necessary phone numbers and the information the Emergency Medical Services (EMS) dispatcher will need to know to send an ambulance. Post a copy of your EIS sheet next to all the phones in the house and office and place a copy in your first aid kit. Make sure everyone at work and in the house, including children, babysitters and caregivers, are familiar with the numbers and how to call for help.

📞 EMERGENCY PHONE NUMBERS

Family Name _____

Address _____

🚑 EMERGENCY: _____

FIRE: _____

POLICE: _____

CALL 911
POLICE · FIRE · MEDICAL
EMERGENCY

☠ POISON HELP: <u>1-800-222-1222</u> _____

🏥 ER / HOSPITAL: _____

DOCTOR: _____

℞ PHARMACY: _____

RELATIVE: _____

NEIGHBOR: _____

WORK: _____

WE'LL BE AT: _____

_____

Make sure all your phone directories (work, home, cell) include the entry ICE (In Case of Emergency). ICE contact is the person you want EMS to call if you're ill or injured. Make sure your children's phones contain an ICE entry, too! Emergency personnel are trained to look for this entry on your cell and home phone when they need information. Your ICE contact should be familiar with your medical history and have access to a copy of your current medical documents.

During a medical emergency, someone should be available to relay instructions if the emergency is not near a phone. It's also a good idea to check the victim for medical information jewelry and to report findings to the dispatcher. Remain calm and listen carefully—the dispatcher may give you valuable first-aid instructions for aiding the victim until help arrives. Pre-arrival instructions over the phone are 'just in time' education, step-by-step actions for CPR and other needed actions. Almost all 911 call centers have this ability. Please, stay on the phone until the dispatcher says it is okay to hang up.

When you call for help, be ready to provide the following information:

- Your name
- Your location
- Description of the emergency
- Number of persons ill or injured
- Your phone number

2. Stock Your First Aid Kit and Your Medicine Cabinet

FIRST AID KIT CHECKLIST

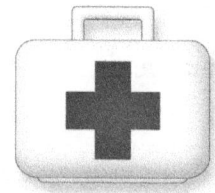

Every home, office and car should have a first aid kit. Make sure everyone knows where it is and what it contains. Below is the First Aid Kit Checklist found in **Doc's First Aide Guide**. Commercially available kits are a good place to start but may   not contain many items you could need. You can use the list below to make your own kit, using a small toolbox or plastic airtight container. Make sure the kit is clearly labeled. Restock it after using and check it regularly to make sure no supplies are missing or outdated.

- ***Doc's First Aid Guide*** with completed EIS

<u>**Equipment**</u>
- CPR barrier mask (face shield)
- Cotton swabs
- Instant activating cold pack
- Paper cups
- Space blanket
- Thermometer
- Sealable Plastic bags
- Battery operated radio

Medication

- Antiseptic wipes/towelettes
- Sterile eye wash with eye cup
- Antiseptic/anesthetic spray
- Antibiotic ointment
- Calamine/antihistamine lotion
- Activated Charcoal tablets/powder
- Wound Saline Wash/Irrigation
- Nalaxone Nasal

Instruments

- Tweezers
- Blunt tipped
  scissor Bulb
  syringe

Miscellaneous

- Disposable gloves
- Candles, waterproof matches
- Pocket flashlight
- Paper/pencil
- Packet tissues
- Soap
- Safety pin

Dressings

  Sterile cotton ball
- Sterile eye patches
- Sterile gauze pads '4x4'
- Hypoallergenic adhesive tape
- Elastic bandage 3 inch
- Roller bandage
- Sterile non-stick pads
- Absorbent compress
- Adhesive bandage strips
- Triangular bandage
- Butterfly bandages

MEDICINE CABINET CHECKLIST

Remember to ask about allergies before giving medication

A well-stocked medicine cabinet will also come in handy in a medical emergency. If you call your doctor's office or insurance company for guidance you may be advised to start treatment at home. Here is a list of items that should be kept in your medicine cabinet, out of reach of young children, of course.

- Acetaminophen, liquid or caplets
- Ibuprofen liquid or caplets. Use for adult fever and as an anti-inflammatory for minor pain.

- Activated Charcoal Tablets/powder. Use for accidental poisoning to absorb toxins/poisons.

- Antihistamine, such as diphenhydramine (generic for brand name 'Benadryl®'). Use for allergic reaction, itching.

- Decongestant nasal spray. Use to clear nasal passageways. Saline nasal spray is a good choice. It is your safest option because you can't use too much and it has no side effects.

  - *NOTE: Be sure to follow directions if you use over-the-counter or prescription decongestants, or combination decongestant /antihistamines. Common ingredients in decongestants, like pseudoephedrine, can affect your heart and blood pressure.*

- Antiseptic antimicrobial liquid for cleaning skin wounds, such as Hibiclens®.

- Thermometer. Use to take body temperature. You should also keep a thermometer in your First Aid Kit. Choose one that is easy to use and interpret. You want to be sure both teenagers and the elderly can use it.

- Expectorant. Use to thin mucus so you can cough it out. Non-prescription Guaifenesin is a good choice

- Cough Suppressant. Use to control your cough. Non-prescription dextromethorphan (DM) is a common ingredient.

- Anti-bacterial ointment. Use after cleaning minor cuts and abrasions. Again, this is included in your First Aid Kit but should also be kept in your medicine cabinet. Bacitracin® is a good choice. Triple antibiotic skin cream contains Neosporin® which is particularly sensitizing, especially when used on the face. It can also cause allergic reactions in some people.

- Calamine or antihistamine lotion, with or without 1% hydrocortisone (HC) are available over OTC. Use this for itching and rash caused by poisonous plants or insect bites. Cleanse the area before application.
- Sterile eye wash with eye cup. Use to flush irritants from eye. You should also keep one in your First Aid Kit.

Check for expiration dates and discard any expired medications properly! Your physician may suggest particular items for your condition.

3. Learn First Aid and Read Your First Aid Book!

It's important to have a current, easy-to-use first-aid book readily available, like *Doc's First Aid Guide*. And please, read it before you need it! Be familiar with what's inside and the steps necessary for basic first aid care.

Understand, however, that reading a book is no substitute for hands-on training. Contact the American Red Cross, American Safety & Health Institute, National Safety Council or the American Heart Association to inquire about first aid and
cardiopulmonary resuscitation (CPR) training. **Knowledge is power**. The more you know the better prepared you'll be to act quickly and correctly in a medical emergency. Remember, the first rule of first aid is to 'Do No Further Harm!'

Emergency care typically starts at home or in the workplace. That's why you must have a first aid kit, a well-stocked medicine cabinet and information on how to provide basic first aid care. You need to be ready to stop bleeding, wash out an eye, or treat a high fever. Waiting for EMS or the ER staff to start treatment means time wasted and a potentially poorer outcome! Be prepared!

4. Make a Health History Sheet

Highlight this section. Put a big asterisk next to it. When you get to the ER, the nurses and doctors need to know your medical history and what medications you are taking in order to give you the best care. They don't know you so you must be your own advocate. Your personal physician will not be caring for you--- even if you get admitted to the hospital. You will be responsible for providing your health history and list of medications. You will be asked for this information over and over again so you can save time and energy by collecting this information now and updating it as needed. You should have a **Pocket Med Card**, listing current medications and dosages, in your wallet at all times.

Be sure to write and pronounce the information clearly. Is your spelling correct, especially in regards to medication? Is your handwriting legible? If you write like a doctor, consider typing your medication list, using the information on the medication bottles as your guide. When you say you're on Clonidine, which is for high blood pressure, does it sound like you're saying Klonopin® which is for seizures or Colchicine for gout? Amlodipine 10mg is antihypertensive medication but sounds like Amitriptylene 10 mg, which is an antidepressant.

You should keep a folder at home with all your medical history documents, along with a dated summary of your medical history and current medications. Whenever possible, bring a copy of the summary with you to the hospital. It's best to carry a copy in case the information isn't returned to you.

Here's a sample Health History Sheet (Medical History / Medication List):

Name: Mary D. Smith (Include middle initial!)

Date: June 1, 2025 (last updated)

Date of Birth: 1/5/1985

Physician's Name(s)/ phone numbers, (Include area code) Dr. Barry Jones, General Practitioner 401-332-3333; Dr. Lee Stark, cardiologist, 401-523-3343

Insurance Company/ phone number: ACE Insurance, 800-444-1111

In Case of Emergency (ICE) contact person / Phone numbers (Include area code): Don D. Smith, son, 443-323-2333 (home), 443-230-4655 (cell)

Clergy: Rev. Brian Clifford, 401-232-1131

Allergies: Penicillin (rash), Latex (rash), Shellfish/Iodine (anaphylaxis)

Very important!! List all medicine, food, and environmental allergens. If you're allergic to penicillin, describe the type of reaction you had when you took it; for example, penicillin (rash). Allergies to shellfish are important to mention because some contrast dyes used in medical testing contain iodine. Latex allergies are also important to note because latex is used in medical equipment and gloves. Again, specify the type of reaction you had. An upset stomach alone is not an allergic reaction.

Medical History: Hypertension (diagnosed 2019), Insulin-Dependent Diabetes (diagnosed 2020), Heart attack (2022), Diverticulitis, Cancer Left Breast (2018), Hypothyroidism (diagnosed 2005)

SURGERIES: Left mastectomy (2018), Appendectomy (1993)

Implanted Devices: Pacemaker Left Chest Wall (2026)

Remember, if you are being treated for a condition, even if it is well controlled, you still have that condition, so list it! List body parts affected. For example, if you had a mastectomy, specify left and/or right breast. Note on this paper if you have any metal in your body, including implants, shrapnel or implanted medical devices.

Family History: Lung cancer (mother, deceased 1999), Diabetes (father), Hypertension (brother)

You may also be asked about your family's health history. Make a note if anyone in your family has had: diabetes, cancer, hypertension, heart disease, aneurysms, as well as any hereditary conditions.

Current Prescribed Medications:
Two Lasix 20 mg (total 40 mg), twice a day for high blood pressure

Aspirin 81 mg, daily

~~*Fexofenadine HCL, 180 mg, daily for allergies*~~ *(stopped 12/2/2017)*

Simvastatin, 40 mg, daily for high cholesterol

Be sure to note the dose along with how many of each pill you take and how often. For example, if you take two 20 mg doses twice a day, spell it out so there's no confusion. State also what condition do you take the drug – medications for high blood pressure are also given for irregular heart rate. Brand names (®) versus generics names can contribute to the confusion.

Double-check your spelling, pronunciation and the dosing information against the bottle.

See how easy it is to make a mistake: Salagen® 5 mg v. Selegiline 5 mg

Salagen® is prescribed for relief of dry mouth symptoms and glaucoma. Selegiline is prescribed to treat Parkinson's disease or depression. Both products are available in 5 mg tablets!

Over-the-counter (OTC)/Herbal preparations:
Co-Q, Red yeast rice, Vitamin C, Calcium, Gingko

This is important! Your health care team needs to know if you're taking any over the counter (OTC) medications because they, too, have side effects and can interact with other medications. The use of topical sulfa ointments on cuts is a great example. These ointments contain an azo dye, 'aseptil rojo' that can make your urine red! So if you go to the ER because you think you have blood in your urine and you don't tell them about this medication, lots of time and money will be spent trying to figure out what's wrong with you. Another example is the use of red yeast rice which when taken in high doses acts like a statin (class of cholesterol lowering drugs) medication and can cause liver disease and breakdown of skeletal muscle. So tell what you take and how often.

Vaccinations:
Flu Vaccine: (date) 11/1/2025

"Tetanus: 2/3/2019"

Pneumonia Vaccine: 10/20/2025

The medical professionals who treat you will appreciate the time and effort you have spent maintaining your health history information. Believe me, you've gained their respect by helping them do their jobs.

The nurse is going to look at your list of medications and ask you when you last took each. If you are admitted to the hospital, chances are the Hospitalist is going to order the drugs on this list for you, along with medications needed to treat you now. Make sure the list you provide is current and dated! Don't add new medications to the list without deleting the old ones you stopped taking! List if stopped within a month.

In some communities, health history and medication information is kept in the refrigerator and a marker is placed on either an entrance door or refrigerator door, alerting emergency personnel to its whereabouts. You can contact your local fire department or ambulance service to determine if this practice is common in your community and what you can do to participate.

Always Carry With You...

Pocket Medication Card with current medications.

Physicians	Immunizations	
Name: _____	Pneumovax	
Phone: _____	Last dose: _____	**POCKET MEDICATION CARD**
Name: _____	Influenza	
Phone: _____	Last dose: _____	**Personal Information**
Name: _____	Tetanus	Name: _____
Phone: _____	Last dose: _____	Phone: _____
Pharmacies	_____	Allergies: _____
Name: _____	_____	_____
Phone: _____	_____	**Emergency Contact**
Name: _____	_____	Name: _____
Phone: _____	_____	Phone: _____

Medication Record Please include all medications from your physicians, including all over the counter and herbal medications.

Drug Name/Strength	Pill/Dose	Time/Day	Reason for Taking	Date Started	Date Stopped

ECG Strip. If you have a cardiac history, carry a minimized copy of your last electrocardiogram (referred to as an ECG or EKG) in your wallet so it can be compared with current ECGs to evaluate any changes.

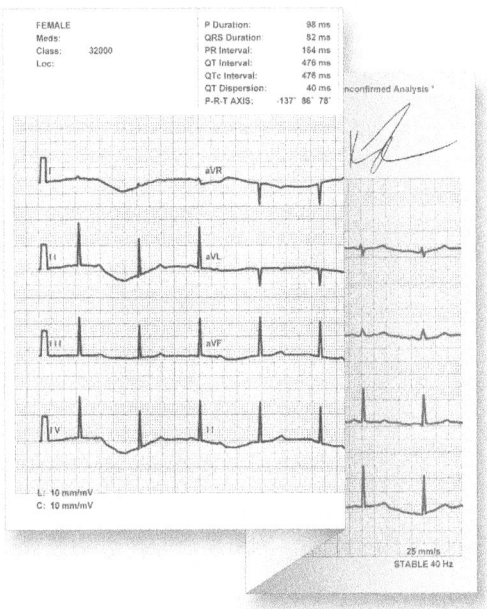

Medical Device ID Cards. If you have a pacemaker or Implantable Cardioverter Defibrillator (ICD), Cardiac Resynchronization Therapy Defibrillators (CRT-Ds) or other medical device, carry a copy of the identification card and any equipment information.

IMPLANTABLE DEFIBRILLATOR
Patient Identification Card

PATIENT	**JOHN DOE**		
	MODEL NUMBER	SERIAL NUMBER	IMPLANT DATE
ICD	**3207-36**	**012345**	**01/JAN/2010**
LV	1058T/86	ABY12345	01/JAN/2010
RVS	7020/65	ABK67890	01/JAN/2010

PHYSICIAN
KATHLEEN A. HANDAL, MD
PHOENIX, AX 85012   PHONE: **602-555-5555**

Medical Jewelry & Health Apps. Consider medical information jewelry (necklace, wrist or ankle bracelet) if you have a medical condition, like diabetes, or are on certain medications, such as anticoagulants! Smartphone Apps abound some are built in, so consider placing medical data for use to help in your healthcare Medical personnel are trained to look for this important information before they treat you.

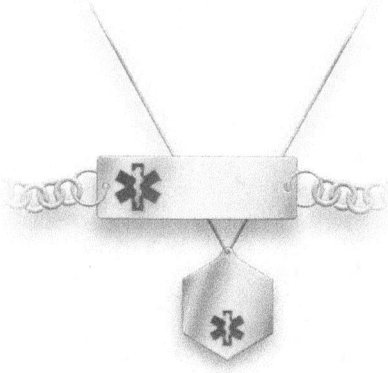

Know Your Blood Pressure ("BP")

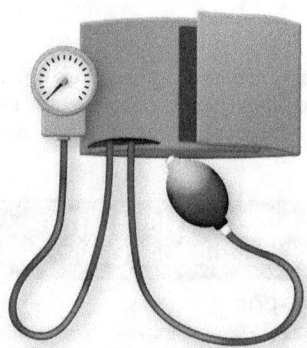

It's also a good idea to know your blood pressure, especially if you have a history of high blood pressure (hypertension). If you have hypertension, you should be keeping a blood pressure log that records A.M. and P.M. blood pressure readings, as well as your pulse. Please bring your recent log with you to the ER! Uncontrolled high blood pressure can kill you, so it is important for you to know what your 'numbers' are and what is normal and abnormal for you.

Date	AM Reading	Pulse	PM Reading	Pulse

Let me explain in general terms what the blood pressure numbers mean: top number (the systolic blood pressure) is the pressure the heart has to overcome to open the valves to pump blood out. Bottom number (the diastolic blood pressure) is the pressure between beats when the heart is resting.

- The "ideal" blood pressure for the average adult is less than 120/80 (120 over 80). High blood pressure is defined as 120/80 or greater. Newer home blood pressure machines have an indicator to alert you when a reading is abnormal. Doctor will set your treatment target blood pressure. Blood pressure typically goes higher with age and activity.

- The normal blood pressure for a 30-year-old is different than the normal blood pressure for a 70-year-old.

- Newer home blood pressure machines have an indicator to alert you when a reading is greater than specific systolic or diastolic. Check your device carefully. Realize a blood pressure reading of 160 over 90 is considered elevated.

- Newer home blood pressure machines also have display detecting motion and 25% deviation from regular heart rhythm, if 'irregular heart beats' are present. This means irregular beats were noted while your blood pressure was being taken.

Your doctor can provide you with information on your normal range and parameters for when to seek medical assistance. If you are on medication to lower your blood pressure you must know what blood pressure readings require you to hold your medication, to take additional medication, as well as when to go to the ER.

- For instance, if your blood pressure is 98/50 should you take your blood pressure lowering medication? The answer is most likely 'no' because lowering your blood pressure any further could be life threatening. In this case, it would be best to call your doctor for advice.

When you monitor your own blood pressure at home, which you must if you are on blood pressure medication, here are some tips to help ensure an accurate reading:

- Avoid caffeine and smoking for 30 minutes prior to taking your blood pressure.

- Sit quietly with both feet flat on the floor for at least three minutes up to five before you inflate the cuff. Do not talk or move any part of your body while machine is recording. It is important to feel relaxed when your blood pressure is taken because stress raises your blood pressure.

- Avoid certain foods and activities prior to taking your blood pressure. Please, don't take your blood pressure after you've gulped down a grande coffee, eaten a meal, or had a bowel movement. A blood pressure reading taken shortly after any one of these actions will be inaccurate. Remember 3 minutes of chilling before taking a reading!

- Always use the arm that has the higher reading, unless there is a medical reason not to, such as an injury, weakness, recent procedure, or breast surgery with lymph node removal.

- If you need to repeat, wait at least two minutes or the second reading may be inaccurate.

Remember: If you are taking blood pressure medication that is not working, as you know it should, get medical help. A blood pressure reading of 180/110 is a medical emergency!

5. Know Your Insurance Coverage

Once an emergency brings you to the ER, the details of your insurance coverage will be secondary to treating your problem. So take the time now to make sure you're carrying a current health insurance identification card. Note your insurance company's contact information on your medical history sheet. Review your policy to find out if any pre-authorization is required and what you must do if you're admitted. Also find out which ERs are covered by your plan and whether the company has a phone help line you can call for advice. Be aware, too, that although your insurance company may approve the ER visit, it may not cover the radiologist, pathologist and even the physician who treated you. Discuss what's covered beforehand with your insurance representative so you aren't surprised when you receive a bill for your visit.

Be aware, too, that you might get a bill from a physician or service whose name you don't recognize. Invoices are often processed through a billing company with a different name. But before you pay the bill, be smart and make sure you are paying for services received.

For more information on health insurance and your rights as a consumer, visit **http://www.HealthCare.gov**. This website, sponsored by the U.S. government, is designed to help consumers navigate the healthcare system.

6. Get Your Legal Documents in Order

It's important to be familiar with the legal documents associated with health care and end-of-life decisions. After all, we are only visitors on this earth! At the hospital, you will be asked if you have advance medical directives, a general term that describes two kinds of legal documents, living wills and medical powers of attorney. Each states' laws vary regarding binding advance medical directives, so it is important to find out the requirements of your state. For more information on these documents, check your state's Health Department and Bar Association websites. They often have the forms you need. For now, here are the basics:

Living Will — Too often people confuse living wills with their personal wills, which describe how they want their assets distributed when they die. They're completely different documents. A living will describes, when you are unable to do so, what type of medical and life-sustaining treatment you expect if you're terminally ill or have been injured and your prognosis is poor. What efforts do you want the medical team to take to prolong your life? That's the main question this document answers. In most cases, you don't need a lawyer to prepare a living will. Some hospitals and physicians provide information on how to prepare a living will. Or you can download a form off the web. Most states require someone to witness your signature. This document does not appoint someone to act on your behalf. That's where the medical power of attorney steps in.

Medical Power of Attorney or Durable Power of Attorney for Health Care — designates a specific person as agent to make healthcare decisions for you when you are unable. Many hospital admitting offices offer you a copy to complete on site. But don't wait until the last minute. Make sure the person you choose understands what type of care you'd expect. You may want a lawyer to assist you with this document.

I recommend that you have advance directives but the decision is entirely up to you. Your ICE contact should have a copy of your advance directives. Better yet, it makes sense to make your ICE contact your Medical Power of Attorney. Advance directives are legal documents. Read them carefully before you sign. Please let family members and your ICE contacts know of your choices in medical matters.

Here are some other healthcare-related legal documents you need to know about:

"Do Not Attempt Resuscitation" (DNAR) — directs health care professionals not to perform cardiopulmonary resuscitation (CPR) if your heart stops beating or you stop breathing. A physician writes this order after a discussion with the patient and his or her family. This is typically assigned when a person is very ill and end-of-life is near and expected. Remember in your living will you can qualify resuscitation efforts and specify that CPR be allowed but not advanced life support (ALS). ALS involves use of drugs and connection to machine(s).

If the order is written in the hospital and the patient goes home or to a nursing home, it's important that the DNAR directive go with the patient so EMS knows how to respond if called. Some states have a color coded DNAR document, making it easy for EMS to recognize. These documents are often posted on the refrigerator so they're easy to find. Check with your local EMS regarding their out-of-hospital DNAR policy.

Uniform Donor Card — indicates to healthcare professionals that you want to donate your organs (ex: eyes, heart, liver, tissue) when you die. It is important to make your wishes known ahead of time by signing a Uniform Donor Card. In most states, you can declare your wishes when you apply for, or renew, your driver's license. Again, be sure your family, ICE contacts and your Medical Power of Attorney know about your choices and intentions.

> *You Need to Know:* When a patient is pronounced dead in the ER, someone from the hospital, typically the ER Charge Nurse, is required to call and report the death to the federally designated, state not-for-profit, organ procurement organization. If the deceased was a donor or can be considered a potential donor, the nurse will then discuss and possibly ask the designated family member to sign a consent form allowing the removal of the organ(s). Everyone recognizes that this is a difficult time for the family. It's important for the deceased's family to remember that other people's lives are on the line and the donation could be a lifesaver for someone else.

Consent to Treat Minors or "Permission to Treat" — names caregivers who have permission to make medical decisions about your minor children when you're unavailable. It is important to have such a document on record at their school. It should describe what medical care can be given in a medical emergency, as well as providing authorization to treat in your absence. Realize that ER staff may not treat without parental consent or such a document unless it is life or limb threatening. Following is a sample consent form:

Consent for Medical/Surgical Care/Emergency Treatment and Child's Medical Information

In presenting my son/daughter for diagnosis and treatment

Name: _____ for _____
    ☐Mother ☐Father ☐Legal Guardian   ☐Son ☐Daughter

of _____ years of age, hereby voluntarily consent to the rendering of such care, including diagnostic procedures, surgical and medical treatment and blood transfusions, by authorized members of the hospital staff or their designees, as may in their professional judgment be necessary.

I hereby acknowledge that no guarantees have been made to me as to the effect of such examinations or treatment on my child's condition.

I have read this form and certify that I understand its contents.

We/I hereby give our(my) consent to _____
                        (Name of Person/Agency)
who will be caring for our(my) child _____
                        (Name of Child)
for the period _____ to _____ to arrange for routine or emergency medical /dental care and treatment necessary to preserve the health of our (my) child.

We/I acknowledge that we are (I am) responsible for all reasonable charges in connection with care and treatment rendered during this period.

Name: _____   Family physician: _____
Address: _____   Pediatrician: _____
_____   Surgeon: _____
_____   Orthopedist: _____
Telephone no.: _____

Name of health insurance carrier: Child's allergies, if any: _____
_____   _____
_____   Date of last tetanus booster: _____
Group no.: _____   Medicines child is taking:_____
Agreement no.: _____   _____

Signature: _____   Date: _____

Witness: _____   Date: _____

In case of emergency I can be reached at:_____
_____

Remember: These are all-important documents and should be readily available in a medical emergency, especially when you're travelling. Copies should be in the possession of your:

- Spouse or Significant Other

- Child's Caregiver (when appropriate)

- Medical Power of Attorney

- ICE contact

- Primary Care Physician / Pediatrician

- Lawyer

These people should also know where the original documents are filed. And always hang on to the original documents. Make copies. Try not to give your original documents to hospital staff because you might not see them again. Once you present a copy in the hospital, it is copied and placed in your file; however, you'll be asked to present it again on the next visit to ensure they have the most up to date information.

7. Get to Know Your ER

Do your homework! You wouldn't dream of buying a car without first checking out the different models, performance, dealerships and their reputations. So why not check out the ERs in your area? After all, not all ERs are the same. Almost every hospital with an ER is accredited by the *Joint Commission (JCJC AHO)*. On site visits are made to evaluate and determine compliance with national standards for quality of patient care and safety. JC accreditation is awarded for three years, except laboratory accreditation, which is awarded for two years. Joint Commission Disease-Specific Care Certification, Primary Stroke Center Certification, and Health Care Staffing Services Certification are awarded for two years.

Besides JC accreditation status, find out if the hospital is a '**Magnet**' hospital this refers to nursing education and staffing ratios. The *American Nurses Credentialing Center's (ANCC)* awards a '**Magnet**' recognition after an on-site visit and evaluation of meeting standards in nursing and patient care. This recognition is reviewed every 2 years.

There are different levels of ERs, also there are specialty medical centers. Here's what you need to know! There are commonly five levels of ERs. The level and title dictates who they are equipped to treat. Level 5 is Urgent Care, Level 4 is rural basic emergency care only.

*Level 1: Highest level ER, indicating the ability to give definitive, rapid care for all critical emergency situations; usually associated with a teaching hospital. Resources within the hospital (diagnostic and intensive care units -ICU) can continue to care for these patients. Level 1 Trauma Centers have an in-house trauma surgeon and on-call specialists available, as well as an open operating room at all times.

*Level 2: The ER can care for most emergencies. All specialties are on-call and available within 60 minutes; usually no residents on staff. EM doctor cares for patient until back-up specialists responds to the request for assistance. In-hospital resources are limited.

*Level 3: Treatment by EM doctors. Not all back-up specialists are available to come to the ER to help. Patient will be stabilized and transported to an appropriate care facility. Trauma patients will be transferred to another hospital that is equipped to handle the trauma

Recognized Specialty centers include:

- Stroke Center: Possible stroke victims should be taken to a Stroke Center, not the nearest hospital. Stroke Centers' ERs are equipped to quickly perform the necessary imaging scans and neurological exams so that clot-busting drugs or clot retrieval can stop or reverse a stroke. Clot-busting drugs need to be given within 3-4.5 hours, or clot removed within 6-16 hours and up to 24 hours of symptoms

- Cardiac Center / Heart Center: Possible heart emergencies, such as heart attack, cardiac arrest (heart stops) and chest pain, should be taken to a Cardiac Center whenever possible. Experienced staff and advanced cardiac resuscitation technology starting in the ER are available here, including cardiac catheterization and hypothermia, both procedures that can help save the heart.

- Pediatric ER: Some hospitals have dedicated pediatric ERs. Great to know if you have children because the staff and facilities specialize in treating children.

- ER with a Fast Track: This type of ER is a good choice if you're suffering from a less-serious illness or injury. Here you're treated by separate staff so there's usually less waiting time.

Now that you know about the different types of ERs, here are some things you can do to learn more about the facilities in your area:

- Use the Internet to find out about the ERs in your area. Most hospital websites describe awards/certifications, the different departments and staff qualifications. Learn if the doctors working in the ER are board certified in Emergency Medicine. Remember, EM doctors specialize in Emergency Medicine, just like cardiologists specialize in the care of the heart. Not all hospitals have this caliber of Emergency Medicine experts on staff. Hospitalists who will also care for the patients when admitted staff some ERs.

- Talk to your doctor and other healthcare professionals and ask for their recommendations.

- Contact your insurance company. It's important to know which hospitals are covered under your plan.

- Visit the different ERs and observe firsthand what they're like. Call in advance, ask for the patient representative or administration office, and schedule a visit. Let them know it will be a quick visit and why you are interested in their facility. Some hospitals may be able to arrange a tour for you. This will give you an opportunity to assess the ER's organization.

- Find out what time the employees change shifts and avoid that time whenever possible because delays are inevitable.

Determine the best routes to the ERs from home and work, taking into consideration the time of day and traffic patterns. Main roads to a hospital are usually marked with a blue sign with a white "H" on it. However, familiarity with back roads is also important, especially if traffic delays are a concern. Learn where to park and where to check in. Areas are usually well marked but familiarity will make finding them much easier.

Remember, EMS has its own criteria for deciding which ER to use. They take into consideration availability, your medical condition and your stated preference. But the priority is always your medical condition! And don't think that calling an ambulance puts you ahead of everyone else in the waiting room. You will be evaluated and seen based on the severity of your injury and illness.

8. Prepare Your Children for the ER

If you have children, consider showing them the ER in your area. Explain what the ER is for and why people go there. This will help to alleviate any fears they might have if they are ever taken there. Visit your library and look for books about emergency care for children, such as *Curious George Goes to the Hospital*. Review your EIS with them. Practice making a 911 call. Make sure they know how to call for help and where the first aid kit is located and how to use it.

*The information covered in **Trauma Run**, a video program Doc Handal produced for children, (K-6) and covers the basic information children need to prepare for a medical emergency and an ambulance trip to the ER. Using a bicycle accident in the desert as an example, it shows children why it is necessary for someone to lay still if a back or neck injury is suspected. It also describes how to call for help, what number to call and what to say to the dispatcher. A small camera was placed on the child victim's head so young viewers could see what it is like from the patient's perspective while being transported to the hospital and examined by a doctor. English and Spanish versions of this program are available.*

Understand that while waiting in the ER, your child may be frightened by the sights and sounds of other injured and ill people. Reinforce that the ER is a safe place where people are helped. Let your child bring a favorite toy to the ER, but not one that makes a lot of noise! Stay calm and provide your child with simple explanations of what is happening and why.

And when your child is being treated, don't say that medicine is candy or that a procedure won't hurt if it will. Calmly describe what to expect and continue to provide comfort and support. Reinforce positive behaviors. Never use the ER or hospital as a threat. Whenever you take a child to the hospital, whether to be treated or as a visitor, remember that hospital floors and other surfaces can carry many germs. Don't let your child crawl on the floor and touch surfaces that may have come in contact with patients. Keep hands and toys clean and away from the mouth, nose and ears!

9. Know When to Go to the ER

How do you know if you need to go to the ER? This is often a tough question to answer. Many factors go the decision, such as the type of injury or illness, signs and symptoms, age and the health history of the person. Hospice patients, for example, shouldn't be taken to the ER unless directed by their physician or nurse. The ER is where you go when something suddenly happens or changes with your body, it is not where you go when you are dissatisfied with your doctor or need a prescription refill.

Some common reasons to seek emergency medical care include:

- Change in alertness or mental status unexplained confusion, loss of consciousness
- Shortness of breath
- Severe headache
- Facial drooping, difficulty speaking or weakness in an arm or leg
- Allergic reaction
- Chest pain
- Bleeding that won't stop with direct pressure

- Severe wounds
- Major injury, such as head trauma
- Burns (area greater than one percent of the body; fingers, toes, genitals, face, neck; third-degree burns)
- Smoke inhalation
- Seizures
- Poisoning
- Severe or worsening reaction to insect bites, medications or foods
- Broken bones
- Coughing or vomiting blood
- Any sudden, severe pain
- Persistent vomiting or diarrhea
- Suicidal or homicidal feelings
- Elevated blood pressure (remember to ask your doctor what is high for you)

Denial can kill! If you're ever unsure whether you're "sick enough" you can always call your primary care physician (PCP) first or your insurance telehealth line. Describe the symptoms and see what he or she advises. Some insurance programs have virtual visit abilities. The doctor may even call ahead and let the ER know you are coming, if necessary.

Like the ER, your doctor's office is a busy place. So have the details of your problem mapped out before you call. The doctor or nurse needs a complete picture of how your body is acting and responding to treatment. Calling and saying "I feel sick" is too vague.

Here's an example of the type of information that paints a complete picture of your problem: *"I noticed a dull pain around my belly button yesterday afternoon around 3 pm. I had no appetite so I didn't eat any dinner. I took two Tylenol PM® at 9 pm and slept for a while. Then I woke with nausea and vomited once around midnight. The vomit was dark, almost black and less than a cup. After I vomited I developed a dull pain in my back and right side. Now..."*

Got the picture?

If your doctor or his office sends you to the ER ask that they call regarding your arrival. Better yet, if you are coming from the medical office ask them to give you something in writing, since they can get busy and forget to notify the ER of your arrival. Take copies of any tests done in the office.

When you're unsure whether or not to go to the ER, calling your insurance company may also be an option. Many insurance programs provide phone help 24/7. Calling this resource is strongly advised by some insurance carriers and may save you time and money. Some programs even provide medical advice over the phone. Don't wait until an emergency occurs to investigate this option. Review your insurance program now and determine what resources are available and what numbers to call. The ER will not know what your insurance covers.

Urgent Care Centers are another option. In fact, your insurance company may direct you to one. Consider going to one for minor illnesses and injuries, such as flu, fever, earaches, nausea, rashes, animal and insect bites, minor bone fractures or cuts requiring stitches. Remember, however, that these facilities may be convenient but are no substitute for hospital emergency care in a medical emergency, such as a heart attack, stroke or trauma. They don't have the same equipment or trained staff as an ER. Many centers conduct physical exams, vision and hearing screenings, and basic lab tests and x-rays. Again, check with your insurance company to learn about the urgent care centers covered under your health insurance policy.

Please don't hesitate too long to get help. It is better to be safe than sorry. I remember a 52-year-old woman who was experiencing what she described as a "feeling" around her chest "like her bra was two sizes too small." She was at work so she decided to wait until her office closed before calling her doctor. When she finally called and told him what she was feeling he ordered her to call "911" so she could get to the hospital right away and to have them call him when she arrived. She said "okay" but after hanging up she wasn't sure if her insurance would pay for the ambulance and decided that driving herself would be quicker. Then she thought about how long she might be in the ER and how unhappy her husband would be if there were nothing to eat when he got home. So she decided instead to release her bra and drive home first so she could have dinner ready for her husband before driving herself to the ER. She eventually arrived at the ER, but with a paramedic on top of her, attempting to revive her. She died in the ER. While driving, she went into cardiac arrest, caused by her heart skipping into a lethal rhythm. This is a sad story of someone who waited too long to call for help and didn't follow her doctor's instructions.

Illness or injury can blur your thinking. Don't drive yourself to the ER. Depending on your situation, call a cab or ask a family member, co-worker or neighbor to drive you. If you are acutely ill or injured, are having trouble breathing, chest pain, or experiencing extreme weakness, call 911/EMS. Life-saving treatment can begin before arriving in the ER.

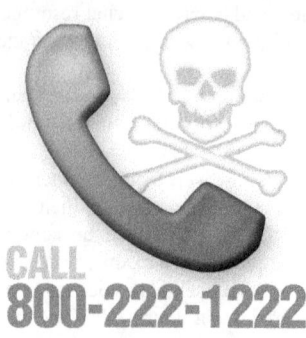

CALL
800-222-1222

In case of accidental poisoning, if time permits, contact the Poison Help Center at 1-800-222-1222. You can dial this number from anywhere in the US, including American Samoa, Puerto Rico, US Virgin Islands and Micronesia. They operate around-the-clock and can provide you with treatment options you can start before reaching the ER.

What can you do when someone refuses medical help?

Convincing a family member or friend that they need to go to the ER is often a challenge. Face it some people are afraid of hospitals, some are just stubborn. Sometimes the illness or injury clouds their judgment. A history of mental illness may also be a factor. You can approach this problem a few ways. You can be blunt and say something like, "Okay, so if you won't go to the ER can I have your car when you die?" Sometimes spelling out the possible consequences convinces people to accept help. You can also contact their physician to see if he or she can intervene. Or you can call 911/EMS and rely on their professional assessment and patient care skills to handle the situation. Always keep your safety in mind in this situation.

10. Get Ready for Emergency Medical Services (EMS)

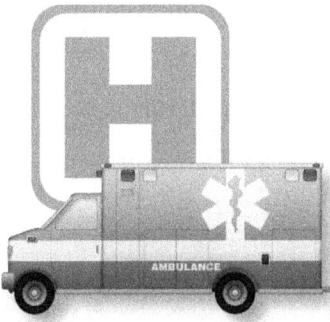

When calling for emergency assistance, be sure to stay on the phone until the dispatcher says it is okay to hang up. EMS may need your help locating the site of the emergency. Please don't call an ambulance thinking you'll be seen faster! That's not the case. As I mentioned before, you'll be triaged along with everyone else and treated accordingly.

You can make EMS's job easier by making your house easy to find in an emergency. Take a good look at your house from the street, the ambulance driver's perspective. Is your house number visible from the road? Is it reflective? Is your walkway clear enough for a stretcher to pass through? Is there a light that can be turned on to illuminate the house and walkway? Is there something that distinguishes your house from the others that will help EMS locate you?

When EMS is on its way, you can prepare for their arrival by locking up pets, securing a clear passageway to the patient, gathering health history and medication information, and sending someone out to the street to help the ambulance driver locate the house. If your house is hard to find, you can blink the porch light to get their attention. Minimize the number of onlookers, as well. One person should stay with the patient and assist with providing information to the emergency personnel. Everyone else should stay clear. If outdoors and a crowd gathers and the patient's privacy is an issue, have a few people stand in front of the victim, facing out, to block the view. Help EMS by answering their questions and staying on the sidelines while they assess the patient.

What's the difference between an Emergency Medical Technician (EMT) and Paramedic?

Emergency Medical Technicians (EMTs) are healthcare professionals who have completed a semester-long training program that prepares them to provide basic emergency medical care to severely ill and injured patients. EMTs have training in CPR, bleeding control, splinting and bandaging, medical emergency care (such as for asthma, diabetes and cardiac problems) and emergency obstetrics. In addition, EMTs can administer oxygen and use a defibrillator.

Paramedics are EMTs who have gone on to attend an extensive, yearlong training program focused on advanced emergency care. Paramedics can establish intravenous lines, place a tube for breathing (intubate), take and interpret electrocardiograms (ECG/EKG), and administer medications. The paramedics are often in radio communication with EM doctors who can advise them on difficult cases or give authorizations for advanced action protocols.

What's Next?

Once inside, the EMTs and/or Paramedics will assess the patient and take vital signs (includes blood pressure). It's important to let them do their work. Telling them to hurry will not help matters. There are steps they have to take before they transport the patient to the hospital. For example, if a spinal injury is suspected, EMS will stabilize the victim's head, neck and back before transporting. Moving a person with this type of injury without stabilizing could result in permanent paralysis. Also some determination of the problem must be made to decide where best to take the patient. In the case of a life-threatening emergency, EMS will take you to the nearest hospital---no matter what your request.

Lights and sirens are only used in certain cases. A safe speed must be maintained to ensure the safety of the patient, the ambulance crew and other drivers. Remember, while en route, care is given by trained medical personnel able to communicate with the receiving hospital ER staff.

Typically, only the parents of young children who are ill or injured are allowed to ride in the ambulance. You'll have to drive to the hospital in your own car. Do not attempt to follow the ambulance. You will be violating traffic rules if you drive above the speed limit or run traffic lights. Drive at a safe speed to the hospital and park in the lot assigned for ER visitors. It's not necessary for everyone in the family to go to the hospital. In fact, it is better if only one or two people are at the bedside. Phone contact between the hospital and home can keep those left behind up to date on the patient's status.

What to Take to the ER

Here's a list of items you should take to the ER — but please use common sense and don't waste time looking for these items in a medical emergency:

- Bucket, if nausea present

- Comfort items, blankets, pillow, teddy bear

- Insurance Card

- Photo ID card

- Copy of Health History Sheet – Medical History / Medication List

- Minimized copy of recent EKG

- Blood Pressure (BP) Log

- Advance Directives, Consent To Treat Minors Documents

- Medical device ID cards and /or manuals

- Medication bottles (if Pocket Med Card is not available)

- Contact numbers / cell phone

- Toys or books for child

- Pen and paper to take notes

- Your ' *Your ER Survival Guide'*

- Hand Sanitizer

- Tissues

More Tips

- Know that ERs can be quite chilly! Last time I was an ER patient the wall clock showed a temperature of 67 degrees, so bring a sweater or jacket. Yes, you can get a blanket but they are usually in short supply.

- Leave patient valuables at home whenever possible!

- If the trip is necessary because of poisoning or overdose, be sure to bring the container for the item ingested, if possible.

- If a body part is severed, place it in a plastic bag and seal it. Then put the sealed bag in cold water and ice and keep it with the owner!

CHAPTER 2

Arriving At The ER

When you arrive by ambulance, EMS will have already notified the ER of your status. Initial treatment will be based on this report. If your condition is critical, you will be treated right away. Don't expect a long meet-and-greet session. The medical staff needs to figure out your treatment plan and doesn't have time for chatting. Friends and family may be asked to wait outside and to assist with registration. It's important to allow medical personnel to do their work, especially if the person is severely ill or injured. If your condition is stable, you may be taken to an assigned area and triaged along with the 'walk-ins'.

If the patient is critical and it is important for you to be at the bedside, let the staff know of your wishes. People do die in the ER, despite optimal and timely care. You should know how to reach clergy when death is expected.

When you are able to walk into an ER, go to the main desk and say why you are there. The receptionist will ask you to fill out a short form with the time (there are clocks everywhere), your name and a brief description of the medical emergency.

Dependent on your condition, you may be taken back into the ER or be directed to the triage area if there is not another patient already there. Don't ever tell anyone "all I have is a cut finger, why can't someone just look at it?" This shows you do not know how the ER works. I'll discuss triage in more detail later on, but understand that a Triage Nurse will speak with you to determine whether or not you need to be seen right away. This mini exam may include your vital signs---temperature, blood pressure, heart rate, respiratory rate and oxygenation level. If you are in pain, you will be asked to describe the pain in your own words and to use a pain scale to rate the intensity of your pain. I'll explain more about pain scales later on.

If you are coughing, you'll be given a mask to wear until you are examined. You will also be asked if you are being controlled or hurt by someone. Hospitals are required by law to ask these questions to help determine if someone is in an abusive relationship. If you are in an abusive relationship, this is a good opportunity to seek assistance.

INSIDE TIP: While ERs are unpredictable, a general guide is to expect the busiest time to be around 6 P.M. As you might guess, 3 A.M. to 9 A.M. is typically quieter, but remember in the ER you cannot predict waiting time. Mondays are usually the busiest day of the week.

If you are taken back into the ER your personal information will be taken when there. An ID bracelet must be issued. Someone will roll in a computer and ask your personal details. '*The American Recovery and Reinvestment Act*' or '**ARRA,**' mandates all patients have electronic medical records (EMR).

If there is a long wait in triage or to get back into ER and you're condition allows you will be registered while waiting. This is when you may need to have your insurance card and ID information ready, as well as information on advance directives. Be sure to use the exact name and address that is on file with your insurance company. The Registrar at the desk doesn't need to know your health history - always know who you are talking to. This person is starting the file (EMR/chart) on you that will follow you throughout your visit. You will encounter a 'PFA' (Patient Financial Advisor) at some point during your visit. If all your information is not complete by the time you are medically discharged you will be asked to stop in their area. You can ask this person questions regarding the financial aspects of your ER visit.

THIS IS IMPORTANT: Your name and date of birth will be used to identify you so make sure they're entered correctly. Even getting your middle initial wrong could put your safety at risk so be sure the registrar got it right. Your health care team will be asking you to repeat your name and date of birth often. Don't get annoyed. Be thankful they're taking steps to make sure they're treating the right person.

A wristband with your name, date of birth, date of admission, and hospital identification number (ID) will be applied, if not already done at triage. Hospitals also apply a second "Allergy Alert" band if you have any allergies. You will be asked to verify the information on the ID band by initialing it before it is put on your wrist.

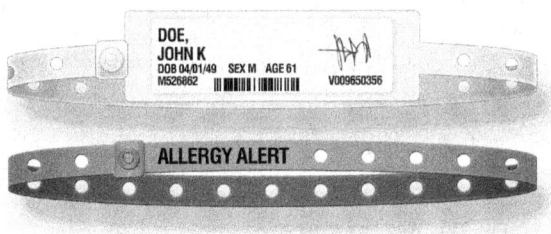

Ask to have the wrist bands placed on your dominant arm because if you need an intravenous line (IV), you'll want the IV in your non-dominant arm.

Remember, ID bands are applied with your safety in mind. Don't remove them. Don't let anyone else wear yours. Once you leave the hospital, these bracelets should be cut up and destroyed like you would an old credit card.

An ER visit isn't free. Expect at some time to be asked for a photo identification card, insurance card and information on your residence and place of work. If you don't have insurance, understand that ERs have a federal directive under the

Emergency Medical Treatment and Active Labor Act (EMTALA) to screen and stabilize patients to determine if the problem is a medical emergency, regardless of their ability to pay. Language from EMTALA:

"In the case of a hospital that has a hospital emergency department, if any individual... comes to the emergency department and a request is made... for examination or treatment for a medical condition, the hospital must provide an appropriate medical screening examination within the capability of the hospital's emergency department, including ancillary services routinely available to the emergency department to determine if an emergency medical condition exists"

The definition of 'emergency medical condition' is also provided under this statute as:

"A medical condition manifesting itself by acute symptoms of sufficient severity (including severe pain) such that the absence of immediate medical attention could reasonably be expected to result in --placing the health of the individual (or, with respect to a pregnant woman, the health of the woman or her unborn child) in serious jeopardy, serious impairment to bodily functions, or serious dysfunction of any bodily organ or part, or with respect to a pregnant woman who is having contractions – that there is inadequate time to effect a safe transfer to another hospital before delivery, or that the transfer may pose a threat to the health or safety of the woman or her unborn child."

This law furthermore prohibits hospitals from delaying your screening examination or care to find out about your ability to pay. If you don't have insurance and are concerned about how you're going to pay for the visit, you can mention it and discuss with the PFA in the ER. Information on assistance may be available. But don't expect any counseling or answers on this topic from the ER Registrar. You can get assistance once your condition is determined. Your priority now is to be examined and treated.

Keep in mind, too, that identity theft is a problem in hospitals. People without citizenship or insurance may try to use your name and insurance information to access health care. Be careful with your personal identification information. Share it only with people who need to know.

Speaking of need to know, you should become familiar with the *Health Insurance Portability and Accountability Act of 1996* (HIPAA). It is a federal law enacted to protect your privacy. Understand that the information put in your file during your hospital visit is only accessible to people who need to know about you, including your health insurer. So tests, lab reports, doctor's notes, and even conversations you have with the doctors and nurses are confidential. This law also gives you the right to access your health record. If you determine incorrect information has been included in your file, there are steps you can take to ask for corrections.

Sounds great, but there's a flip side, should someone call the ER to find out how you're doing, no one can tell them you're there or how you're doing without your permission. You will be asked to specify who may medical staff talks to about your status.

Remember that pen and paper I told you to carry? Start taking notes upon arrival to the ER. Use your Smartphone if necessary. This is for your own reference. A trip to the ER is stressful and it's easy to miss important information so keep a log of events. Note the names of the people caring for you; what tests were run, the diagnosis, medications and treatment. Time can go slowly and you might think it has been an hour since your blood test, yet when you look at your notes you might see it was done only 25 minutes ago! Remember, you have a right to understand what is being done to you and why. You will be receiving information on your rights as a patient from the hospital staff. The Patient's Bill of Rights is usually posted in the ER. In general, as a patient you have the right to:

- Be treated with respect

- Information and choice

- Privacy

Remember, you have a right to have a test, medicine or procedure explained to you before you receive it. You are free to accept or refuse treatments if you are unclear or not satisfied as to why it was ordered. The ordering staff member, commonly the EM doctor, will be told of your concerns and should approach you to discuss them. The policy requires that you have a detailed explanation of what refusal of treatment means, and to be told what negative effects this may have on your health. You must accept responsibility for refusal to follow the treatment plan. You also have the right to refuse to participate in medical research.

Take responsibility for your health care. Participate in all decisions about your treatment. "It is your body!"

Business Card, Please!

When you meet the EM doctor, hospitalist, social worker, charge nurse or a consulting physician, ask for their business card so you can reach them later on. If they don't have one, write down their name and how to reach them in your handy note pad. And don't forget to thank the people who help you. It will go a long way in making everyone's day brighter, including your own.

Presenting Your Problem

As mentioned earlier, the first medically trained person that you will be evaluated by is the Triage Nurse. Make sure that when this nurse sees you that you clearly describe the problem, using as few words as possible. There's a big difference between "I've got a pain in my arm" and "I have a pain in my left arm, radiating to my back and chest. And I feel short of breath." The first comment will get you a 'number' and a seat. The second will get you immediate entry and a bed. If the problem is serious, and potentially life threatening, you need to make this known.

Here's another example: "I feel kind of tired and lightheaded. I get like this sometimes and then I'm okay" or "I feel weak and lightheaded and I'm a diabetic. My last blood sugar reading was 50." The addition of the word "diabetic" along with your blood sugar reading makes it clear that the problem could be potentially serious. Got the picture? But do not lie in order to be seen quicker, you may end up with a lot of tests or even admitted unnecessarily to the hospital!

- The Triage Nurse will also take your vital signs. It's important to know that your vital signs reveal a lot about your present health status. Certain results will trigger immediate attention. The Triage Nurse may also order tests, based on "standing orders" already in place for certain signs and symptoms. So yes, you can get an ankle x-ray before being examined by the EM doctor when a 'standing order' protocol for ankle trauma is in place. If you have to use the bathroom, ask if a specimen may be needed. If a urine test is likely to be ordered, you'll be given a container and instructions.

- If you are pregnant or could be pregnant, speak up. This information is important. There are imaging studies (x-rays/scans) and certain medications women shouldn't receive when pregnant.

- If you have been treated in the hospital before, whether as an inpatient or in the ER, tell the Triage Nurse so your 'old' medical records can be accessed, if necessary.

Language Barriers

If there are any language barriers, or you feel like you're not being understood, request a translator. Hospitals either have persons on site who can translate or access to a phone translation service. If you are accompanying a non-English speaking person to the hospital and expect to translate, don't be offended if the hospital calls in another translator. Medical professionals often prefer to use their own translators because family members may not repeat the patient's statements word for word and may include their own interpretation.

ID Please!!! Make Sure They've Got the Right Patient

Before anyone touches you or performs a test, make sure they identify themselves and verify your identity by asking your name, date of birth, and/or check your ID bracelet. If someone doesn't take this step, question why (nicely) or offer up your name to make sure you're who they think you are. In addition, ask staff who they are, if they don't tell you first. Everyone who works in the hospital should be wearing a badge and announcing who they are before they care for you. You have a right to know who is taking care of you and what their role is in your care.

Why Are Other People Being Seen Ahead of You?

You've been waiting to be seen for over two hours when you notice that the man who came in ten minutes ago is being taken ahead of you. He doesn't look any sicker than you. You become angry, frustrated and wonder if they've forgotten you. Entitlement mentality is bad in everyday life, and in the ER it is really bad. Remember the Triage Nurse you saw earlier? Well, this nurse is the 'gatekeeper'; she knows who is waiting for beds and what beds are available 'in the back'. There's a system at work. It's highly unlikely, but not impossible, that you've been forgotten. You can go to the front desk and inquire, but first think about the system and where you might fit in.

The Emergency Severity Index (ESI) was designed for ER triage by the US Department of Health & Human Services, to determine who gets medical care and in what order. The ESI is a five-level algorithm that prioritizes patients into five groups from 1 (most urgent) to 5 (least urgent) based on acuity (seriousness) and the resources that person may need. Triage staff use specific criteria to determine each patient's acuity. ESI groups and examples:

1. **Resuscitation** (trauma, cardiac arrest, heart has stopped)
2. **Emergent** (life or limb threatening, chest pain, stroke)
3. **Urgent** (abdominal pain)
4. **Non-urgent** (broken arm)
5. **Referred** (medication refill)

A well-implemented ESI program helps hospital ERs rapidly identify patients in need of immediate attention, and allows them to better identify patients who could safely and more efficiently be seen in a fast track rather than the main ER. This system also allows the hospital to more accurately determine the ER's need to go on 'diversion'; that is, ask that ambulance patients be taken elsewhere as capacity has been reached. This is only done under set situations usually decided by the local EMS system.

"Fast Track" Option

So if your ankle is swollen and the ambulances are rolling in with critical patients, take heart. There may be another system in place for less critical patients like you. Some ERs utilize a Fast Track system where less acute patients are seen. The examination area is different and so is staffing and supplies. So the good news is you might be in and out faster. You can rest assured that if your condition worsens you'll be taken to the main ER. However, delays are still possible. If you need tests, and that includes an x-ray, you might have to wait, even if you are the only person in the Fast Track area. The reason is that some hospitals do not have a dedicated imaging (radiology) department or lab for the Fast Track, so you're in line with the rest of the folks from the main ER. There is usually a copy of the hospital's "Patient Information Booklet" in the waiting areas. Spend your time reading this information---it will empower you!

While You're Waiting...and Waiting

Lack of predictability is the only thing you can count on now. You're probably wondering why someone doesn't come out and at least tell you how much longer it will be until they can see you. Some ERs attempt to share wait time but it is not guaranteed. The truth is, they'd like to be accurate, but they can't. They don't really know. Remember, this isn't a restaurant or technical support hotline. The waiting area may be quiet but the back area is probably hopping.

Ambulance entrances are usually out of sight from the main ER entrance and waiting area. At any moment, a critically ill patient could arrive or the condition of a person already being seen could worsen, requiring the attention of most of the emergency medical staff. At the same time, there's a limit to how many people can be seen at one time, and the people already back there are being treated. You've just got to trust that you'll be called when a spot is available. After all, waiting is good! The person you have to feel sorry for is the one rushed in ahead of you. Standing and staring at staff trying to intimidate them will not get you seen faster. So lighten up! Laugh a little and tell some jokes. It won't make you feel any worse. My saving grace while working in the ER for so many years was my ability to laugh. Sure, the ER is intense and scary, but what better way to cope than to look on the brighter side? Someone might be getting a second chance at life behind those doors!

But if you're getting worse, please make it known. Be specific. If your back now aches from sitting in the chair for so long, that's cheating. But if the pain in your left side has gone from a level "three" to "nine", speak up. If you vomited in the bathroom, don't shout or scream, just let the Triage Nurse know that your condition is changing and you're concerned.

Nothing By Mouth (NPO)!

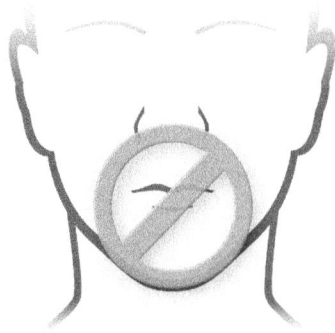

Hungry? Thirsty? Whether or not you should eat or drink depends on why you're there. If the tip of your toe is hanging off, you can probably eat. I say 'probably' because the reason food and drink is discouraged is because some tests and medications require that you have an empty stomach. In addition, if a procedure involves some pain or numbing medications and you react to this cocktail poorly, the hot dog and latte you ate earlier may end up in the emesis (vomit) "EME" bag or basin.

If your problem can't be fixed with a nerve block or local anesthesia (numbing the area to be worked on) you'll be given intravenous (IV) sedation and 'knocked out'. If you have a full stomach while under anesthesia, there's a chance the contents will come up and the vomit could get into your lungs, causing you to aspirate (food/liquid enters the airway). That's why operations and procedures are often delayed. They want to make sure the stomach is empty before proceeding.

If you're in the ER because of abdominal pain or vomiting, you definitely shouldn't eat or drink because you will most likely be having tests that require an empty stomach. The bottom line: If you're hungry, ask the Triage Nurse for advice. If a long stay is expected, it will be up to your doctor to determine whether and what you can eat.

The dietary term assigned to someone who is not allowed to eat or drink anything, including ice chips, is NPO. Where did the term NPO come from? "N" stands for "nil" which you know means 'nothing' and "per os" is Latin for "by mouth". Thus, NPO means NOTHING by mouth, no exceptions. Some doctors will order: "NPO except for ice chips and medications." Or they'll order "clear liquids" which typically consists of water, Jello™, ginger ale, and Italian ice. Don't cheat. Diet orders are written for a reason. If you're unclear why you're assigned a certain diet, simply ask.

Organize Your Thoughts

Use the waiting time to think about what you're going to tell the nurse and doctor about your situation. Prepare notes that you can refer to when you present your case.

- When did the problem start?

- What were you doing when it started?

- How did you treat it?

- Did the treatment have any effect?

- Did it make it worse?

- Has this happened before? If so, how was it treated?

Keep it short and simple but cover the facts. Forget describing a time when your Aunt Myrtle had a gallbladder attack in 1965 and you took her to the emergency department and had to wait for an hour and she had a fever and maybe that's what you've got… yada, yada, yada.

Instead, focus on you and your immediate problem and say "Doc, at 1:30 today I ate fish and chips at a restaurant. One hour later I developed a sharp pain in my right side. I took an antacid but it didn't help. The pain has been increasing and I vomited a cup of green liquid about an hour ago…" Got the picture? Be sure to mention any health history information related to this current situation, such as irritable bowel syndrome (IBS), or gallstones, or the fact that your gallbladder was taken out last week.

You're Up!

Some ERs are open bays of uncomfortable stretchers (beds), separated only by cloth curtains, making it easier to monitor a large number of patients at one time. The newer ERs have a higher degree of visual and acoustic privacy. Women with possible obstetrical, gynecological or abdominal complaints may be placed in a specially equipped 'Gyn' room. However, there are only a few situations that will get you a totally private room away from the main action.

Critical trauma patients and cardiac resuscitation patients are usually cared for in less visible areas near the ambulance entrance. Depending on the size of the ER, you may also be taken to an area related to your chief complaint. For example, if you have a broken leg you may be placed in an orthopedic area, surrounded by all kinds of crutches and equipment used to treat orthopedic emergencies.

You'll be given a gown to wear. It's likely no one will explain this means you have to take your clothes off before putting this on so we can see and examine the area of your problem. If you are told to stay in bed, do so! You should be told how to call for help. If no one tells you, ask. Remember you are your own advocate.

Because of the layout, you'll probably hear and see things that you can't wait to tell your friends about. Please don't. Remember the saying: "Do unto others as you would have them do unto you." Respect the privacy of those around you. After all, the hospital staff has to respect your privacy---remember HIPAA?

CHAPTER 3
Meet Your Team

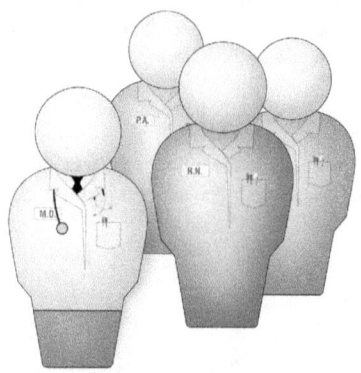

Your Nurse

Most likely, the first person you'll meet in the 'back' is a nurse. He or she has received some basic knowledge of why you're there from the triage report. Many ER nurses are certified in Emergency Nursing. You'll know if your nurse has these credentials if he or she has Certified Emergency Nursing (CEN) or Pediatric Emergency Nursing (CPEN) after their name. Re-examination and continued education is required to maintain these credentials. They are excellent lie detectors, so do not lose credibility---tell the truth!

An ER nurse is responsible for:

Monitoring vital signs — Remember this includes heart rate, blood pressure, respiratory rate, temperature, and pain level. Initially we're looking to see if the numbers are too high or too low and whether something has to be done right away to correct the problem. For instance:

- If your heart rate is 150 (which is high for an adult) we're going to have to quickly determine why and treat the problem.

- If your blood pressure is too low, say 60/40, we're going to have to establish the cause and either give you medication or IV fluids to raise your blood pressure.

- If your breathing is shallow we'll try to uncover the reason and take steps to correct the problem.

- If your temperature is elevated, we'll look for the cause while attempting to bring it back to normal.

- In certain cases, oxygenation is also monitored, as part of your respiratory assessment. Usually a clip device is attached to your fingertip. If your oxygen saturation (SaO2) is low, let's say at or below 88 percent, or your condition is urgent, serious, oxygen will be given through your nose or a mask.

NOTE: While there are guidelines for what is considered "normal" vital signs, each of us is unique. Our age, weight and medical conditions factor into what is best for us and what is out of bounds! Therefore, the next time you see your medical provider ask what your 'normal' is and include this information on your health history sheet.

Using the Pain Scale

Pain is considered the fifth vital sign. Here's when you get your lesson on using the pain scale, a system for determining your level of pain and whether or not it is being well controlled. There are different types of pain scales but the most commonly used one has a numerical rating scale. Here's how it works. The nurse will ask you:

"On a scale of one to ten, with ten being the worst pain ever and one almost none, how would you rate your pain right now?" There is no right or wrong answers so say whatever you are feeling. However, this is not the time to try to get more attention by exaggerating your pain level because it could land you in the operating room! Minimizing it might get you there, too, so be honest and straightforward. Understand, too, that pain may not be treated until a working diagnosis of your complaint is established.

If the nurse gives you pain medication for a pain level you rated as "seven", she's going to check back with you later on to see how well the pain medication worked. If the level is the same or hasn't changed much, this indicates to your nurse that additional pain medication may be needed. If you rate your pain as "one" and say you feel much better, she knows the pain medication worked. But that's not the end of it.

You'll be asked regularly to report your pain level number. Again, this is done for your comfort and safety and to decide the best care, so please cooperate. The nurse will be documenting the time with your responses. This helps to determine if your condition is changing and how much pain medication you may need and how often. It also helps to identify when a type of pain medication isn't working and when another one should be ordered.

Children, elderly or anyone who may be confused may be asked to express their pain level using visual aids. This type of scale provides a visual description of pain for those who are unable to verbally communicate their discomfort. By acknowledging or pointing to the image that best matches how they feel, the patient provides the nurse with a good sense of how much pain they're experiencing.

Conducting a physical and mental assessment — Your nurse will examine you in relation to your problem but also monitor for other potential problems that could develop, based on your illness or injury. Your mental status is also being evaluated. Answer questions appropriately. Your nurse doesn't know you and may misread, in the wrong way, any attempts at humor.

Gathering your health and medication history — You'll make an immediate friend when you present your Health History Sheet and your Pocket Med Card. If you remember to state when you last took your medications you'll get a gold star. This is the time, again, to repeat what happened and why you came to the ER. The nurse is going to write it all down so be thorough and concise. Make sure your nurse knows about any allergies, as well. No one wants to give you anything that's going to trigger an allergic reaction. Do not forget your OTC and herbal treatments.

Developing a plan of care — Based on your signs and symptoms, the nurse and the EM doctor will develop a plan of care for treating your problem. This might include monitoring urine output, continuous cardiac monitoring, bed rest, nothing to eat or drink, to name a few. Your nurse is the person to ask if you are unclear, or haven't been told, about such things as whether you can get out of bed, eat, or use your cell phone.

Administering medication — Your nurse is responsible for giving you medication, following the five RIGHTS of safe medication administration: Right patient, right medication, right dose, right time, and right route. Your nurse should ask you your name and date of birth and check your bracelet to make sure you're the right patient before giving you any medication. Understand that in an emergency that is life or limb threatening these actions are subtle.

TIP: It is best to lie down when your nurse gives you a shot, even if the shot is in your arm. Lying flat also helps to distribute the medication more effectively into your system. If you're right handed and the nurse wants to give you a shot in the arm or start an IV, ask to have it in the left arm. If you know where you have a good (easy) vein to access, whether for an IV or drawing blood, speak up! This will make it easier for you and the technician or nurse.

Communicating with the EM Doctor — If you develop nausea, increased pain, weakness, anything new, the nurse will let your EM doctor know and get orders for what to do to handle the problem or situation. Understand that the nurse can't give you any medication without an order from the doctor.

Monitoring test results — The nurse and the EM doctor will be watching for test results with the help of the ER support staff. Most ER records are now electronic and this helps to expedite care. When told results, be sure to note them on your pad so you'll have your own record. Should a consultant incorrectly state a test result, you'll be able to set the record.

Communicating with you — You need to know how to reach the nurse if you have needs, so ask early on how to get help. Understand, too, that your nurse has other patients, is working either an 8 or 12-hour shift and has to go home at some time, so you may have more than one nurse. Get to know your nurse(s) by name and work with them to get the best care possible. You are your best advocate!

Preparing for discharge — From the moment you arrive, the nurse is preparing for your eventual discharge – no one stays in the ER indefinitely. Once the EM doctor decides where you're going next, your nurse will execute the order and handle whatever paperwork and review your instructions. If you're admitted to the hospital or transferred, your nurse will make sure information about your admission is sent to the next nurse.

EM Doctors

Now we're going to talk about a topic near and dear to my heart, the role of the EM doctor.

The doctor who sees you in the ER is most likely a specialist (Board Certified) in Emergency Medicine. They work closely with other specialists and will contact your primary care physician (PCP), when necessary, in order to give you first-rate care. Board Certified EM doctors have passed a comprehensive exam administered by a certifying Board of Emergency Medicine. My specialty also requires yearly self-assessment tests and recertification every 10 years. Trust me, Board Certified EM Docs know Emergency Medicine!

Every physician working in an ER, whether or not they are Board Certified in Emergency Medicine, has certain responsibilities, which include:

Evaluating Your Condition — The EM doctor will ask you about your problem and then examine you to determine what might be wrong. I say, "might" because this initial exam may only provide what we refer to as a "differential diagnosis". Not all cases are straightforward, like suturing a deep cut or repositioning a dislocated shoulder. Tests, or maybe a second opinion, may be necessary to confirm a diagnosis. So do not withhold information or a diagnosis that you have already received from your PCP just to see if we come up with the same ones. All you are doing is slowly down your care. The focus is on the problem you reported and all potential ramifications. Your diagnosis may not be made until after all test results are back.

Keep in mind that your visit to the ER may not identify or solve your problem. For some, time is needed to reveal what the exact problem is and/or the extent of it. The proverbial tip of the iceberg! You may not leave the ER with a definite diagnosis;

however, the EM doctor will have determined that it is safe for you to go home and refer you for further testing and evaluation as an outpatient.

TIP: Don't talk while anyone is listening to your heart and lungs with a stethoscope. We can't hear when our ears are plugged. Wait till we're finished to talk, please. If you want to help, loosen clothing so the stethoscope can be brought to touch bare skin from which we can hear best. Now is not the time to be modest.

Again, the EM doctor has been told why you are there but will also be asking you to describe your problem. I know this gets tiresome but it is your story and it is best when we hear it from you. When asked what's wrong, stick to the facts. Refer to your notes. And tell the truth. Doctors are great detectives. We can usually tell if your story doesn't make sense or you're leaving something out. So tell all! What you say is confidential and will help you get the appropriate care as quickly as possible.

About Alcohol and Substance Abuse

People tend to minimize the amount of alcohol they consume. If you drink six beers a day, say so. Don't say you drink a beer or two once in a while. Alcohol affects your body in many ways. If you drink on a regular basis and are rushed to the operating room you could die if the anesthetist does not know about the extent of your drinking. If you are admitted to the hospital, you may experience withdrawal symptoms that will complicate your condition. There is always a first time. So tell us in order that medication to help is given.

Also be honest about your drug use, both street and prescription. Narcotic withdrawal, whether from street heroin or Percocet, can tremendously complicate any illness. Know that certain therapeutic medications don't sit well with street drugs and opioids and may even result in adverse effects – so tell the truth!!

If you smoke, tell the doctor. Most likely, you're not going to be able to go outside for a smoke while you're being seen. The EM doctor can order a nicotine patch for you that should help with your cravings. Smoking in a hospital is a serious offense. Oxygen is in use and can ignite when exposed to open flames from matches or cigarettes. In some hospitals, violators of the no smoking rule will be prosecuted.

Ordering tests and blood work — Depending on your problem; tests may have already been started before the EM doctor physically sees you. This may mean that the EM doctor was alerted by the nurse of your condition or that standing orders related to your complaint and vital signs were followed. If your care involves going to the operating room, blood tests will be necessary and possibly an ECG. An explanation of some of the common tests that may be ordered can be found in Chapter 4.

Understand that test results are not always positive or negative. The EM doctor has to evaluate the results in the context of what brought you to the ER, your complaints, and vital signs as well as how you feel at the moment. Even a positive pregnancy test can be open to interpretation, depending on the situation presented.

Understand, too, that the testing process can take time. Viral and other unique lab tests may need to be sent out to a specialty lab or even an out of state lab. Some test results, like cultures that identify a specific type of bacterial infection, can take two days to develop. And sensitivity results, which help to identify the appropriate antibiotic to use to kill the bacteria, are usually only available after two days of culture growth. So if other signs and symptoms and test results point to a possible bacterial infection, you'll be treated with an empiric (best guess) antibiotic. The antibiotic ordered for you, as the culture is taken, may have to be changed once the type of bacteria is identified. Or if there is no evidence of a bacterial infection, you might be told to stop the antibiotic.

TIP: Don't bother to ask for routine exams like your Pap smear or prostrate exam or to have your prescriptions refilled. Now is not the time to deal with these issues. We're focusing on the problem that brought you into the ER.

Ordering Medication — The medication ordered is based on your current complaint and diagnosis, as well as your medical history. This is where an accurate list of medications and problems you have, or have had, are important. If you are a diet-controlled diabetic and take no medication the doctor needs to know!

Discovery — Based on your exam and your test results, a determination of the most likely diagnosis will be made and the appropriate medical care plan will be created. Some patients will have no clue as to how close they came to dying before being saved by emergency treatments. Bragging is not allowed in the ER---it's our job to save lives! My motto is 'when you hear hoof beats don't just think of horses – think zebras'! That's why often an unusual diagnosis missed by others is made in the ER.

Call your personal physician — Be sure to have contact information for your personal physicians available so the EM doctor can call him or her with any questions or concerns. Transmission of your records is easy in this age of technology.

Order consults — When your condition is unclear, or is so complicated that immediate care by another specialist is warranted, a call will go out to either a specialist of your choice or the on-call physician for that specialty. Hospitals are mandated to have specialty resources available to back up the EM doctors. Often a phone consult is all that is needed. But if the specialist needs to see you, you might have to wait a while because they seldom work in the ER. However, this might not be the case if you're in a teaching hospital where specialists are more likely to be readily available. Here it is likely a resident will initially see you, rather quickly, whom the attending physician of the service will supervise.

Physician Assistants (PAs)

Physician Assistants, commonly referred to as "PAs", can function in a similar role as the EM doctor. However, their licensed roles may vary from state to state. One difference between them and the MD or DO doctor is their education; a PA degree is a two-year program versus at least an eight-year program (after college) for the EM certified doctor. Certified PAs will have PA-C after their names. PA-Cs are required to log Continuing Medical Education (CME) 100 hours every two years and pass a recertification exam every ten years. Each state and hospital sets parameters for physician 'supervision' of PAs but typically they work under the supervision of the doctor on duty in the ER. PAs can prescribe medications in all states. They may see and treat patients but confer with the doctor as necessary. You can always request to talk with the EM doctor if you feel your needs aren't being met by a PA.

Residents

If you go to a teaching hospital's ER expect to be greeted by at least one resident. If you are an interesting case, guaranteed you'll have a crowd of them circling around you. They're typically very keen and current on the latest treatments. Residents have completed four years of medical school and one year of internship and are supervised by an Attending Physician. They become licensed physicians after a one-year internship. Residency is specialty training above and beyond what is required to be a licensed doctor. The residency gives in-depth training within a specific branch of medicine, and the number of years spent as a resident varies according to specialty. Residents might be in training for Emergency Medicine if the institution has an approved program.

Interns and Medical Students

ERs are training grounds for interns and third-and fourth-year medical students. They're supervised by on-site EM Attending Physicians. Remember, tomorrow's doctors have to start somewhere, so be patient. If you're unsure whether you're getting the necessary treatment, you can always ask to be seen by the Attending!

Nurse Practitioner (NP) and Advanced Practice Registered Nurse (APRN)

"NP" or "APRN" (a specific type of NP) after a nurse's name denotes a licensed advanced practice nurse. After certifying as an RN, they continue to advanced education and clinical training. They have years of education: a four-year Bachelor of Science in Nursing, plus an additional two-year Master of Science in Nursing. They are licensed by the state and many practice in specialty and sub-specialty areas of medicine.

They have years of education: a four-year Bachelor of Science in Nursing, plus an additional two-year Master of Science in Nursing. They are licensed by the state and many practice in specialty and sub-specialty areas of medicine. There are over 30,000 in the U.S. and, at this writing, in 34 states. They can write prescriptions; nurse practitioners require no physician supervision. They are commonly found in medical office settings, and also as part of the Fast Track and ER teams.

Hospitalists

If a decision to admit you is made, a Hospitalist group of doctors will be taking care of you during your stay. Insurance companies contract with medical groups to provide in-hospital care. They are assigned to work in the hospital and are very familiar with hospital procedures and services. Often, they are Internal Medicine specialists who will coordinate with other specialists caring for you. When you are discharged you will go back to being under the care of your PCP. Gone are the days that your personal physician can care for you while you are in the hospital.

Phlebotomists

Most hospitals have phlebotomists; they're the folks who draw the blood and make up the IV team. They're experts at what they do because they do it all the time. In some hospitals, nurses or technicians perform this role, as well. The phlebotomist will assess your arms, looking for a good vein to access. Volunteer a good vein if you know you have one. Finding a good vein may take some time, depending on your age, general health and hydration status. If you're elderly, ill or dehydrated your veins may not be easy to locate. A pocket transillumination device might be used to help locate a vein. Or, the phlebotomist, after tying a band (tourniquet) around your upper arm, will finger tap the veins, or perhaps apply warm compress. (This is also done when inserting an IV.) Once the vein is accessed and blood is flowing, how many vials of blood are taken depends on the lab tests ordered.

Critical patients have a 'rainbow' drawn---you guessed it, a vial for every color! Different colored tubes indicate different tests. You can always ask the phlebotomist which labs are being drawn. Realize that most tubes are filled by less than a teaspoon of blood! When the needle is removed, apply pressure to the site to stop the bleeding. If you've been on aspirin or blood thinning medication, like Coumadin® (warfarin), you may need to elevate your arm and apply pressure to stop the bleeding. Leave your bandage on while in the ER, it will remind all that you had blood drawn.

If a vein is 'blown', that is when the needle goes through two sides of your vein, blood will leak into the skin, and you'll see the start of a bruise. It's important to apply pressure, elevate the site and apply a cold pack immediately. Markings from blood draws can last a week, especially if there is bruising and swelling at the site.

Transporters

Transporters take you via wheelchair or stretcher to fun places like the imaging department (radiology) or, if you're lucky, to your car. The transporter should check your identification to make sure you are the right patient before you go anywhere. It's important for you to ask where you are being taken and for what purpose (test). If you're being taken to surgery and you're in the ER for an asthma attack, please ask to see your nurse. Mistakes happen.

Also make sure you're comfortable because you may be in the wheelchair or on the stretcher for a long time as you travel to parts of the hospital you never knew existed. If you're cold, ask for a blanket. If you can't breathe when you lie flat, ask to have your head elevated. Let the transporter know if you need to use the bathroom. If you have any valuables with you, leave them with family or friends because you might not be able to take them into the testing area. If you're alone, you can ask the nurse to ask hospital security to lock up your valuables.

CHAPTER 4

Studies & Procedures

Time to Talk about Diagnostic Testing

A visit to the ER wouldn't be complete without some type of test. Following is a simplified overview of some of the basic tests you might encounter.

Interpreting Blood Tests

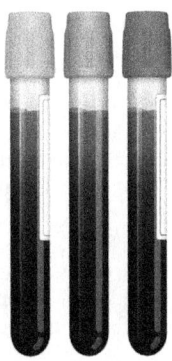

It's impossible to explain every blood test and what it means in the context of this book. My recommendation is to write down the names of the tests that are ordered on you and to ask the EM doctor what the results mean. Diagnostic tests are not always positive or negative. The findings must always be evaluated in the context of what was abnormal in your examination and why you are in the ER. Understand, too, that sometimes the results and the answers aren't immediate.

Complete Blood Count (CBC) — You've heard it ordered on the TV shows, "Get me a CBC stat!" STAT comes from the Latin "statim" meaning immediately. A CBC is a common blood test that provides a general picture of your blood levels. It's typically ordered for complaints such as fatigue, weakness, inflammation, bruising, fever and bleeding. It is an automated count of the cells in your blood that includes information on the number, shape and size of your cells. A standard CBC includes eight tests, with the big five being:

White Blood Cell (WBC) — count helps to identify infection, immune problems, cancer and leukemia. If the numbers are high or low, further testing is usually required.

Red Blood Cell (RBC) — count helps to identify anemia if decreased.

Hemoglobin (HGB) — measures the oxygen-carrying proteins in the blood. When low, it can indicate anemia, which may be due to several causes including blood loss, vitamin or iron deficiency, and cancer. Severe anemia can be life-threatening.

Hematocrit (HCT) — measures the percentage of red blood cells in a given volume of blood. Again, if the level is low, anemia is indicated.

Platelets — identify problems related to bleeding and clotting.

Next up in the "ER" list of frequent tests on blood is the Basic Metabolic Panel (BMP) which checks the electrolyte and mineral levels that are so important for keeping your muscles, heart and other organs working properly. Included here is your level of:

Sodium (Na), — which is important for regulating the fluid balance in your body and transmitting electrical signals in the brain and muscles. When you're dehydrated, due to vomiting or diarrhea, your level could be high or low. Signs of a sodium imbalance are confusion, weakness and lethargy. IV medication is necessary to correct the imbalance.

Chloride (Cl) — also helps to regulate fluids in your body. Chemical reactions are taking place in your body at all times. When a chemical like chloride is lacking, the blood becomes more acidic and reactions don't occur efficiently and your body doesn't function properly.

Potassium (K) — is necessary for proper functioning of heart rhythm and plays a key role in skeletal and smooth muscle contraction. If your level is too high or too low, you're at increased risk of abnormal heartbeats. Muscle weakness is often related to a low potassium level. A low potassium level is often the result of: diarrhea, vomiting, excessive sweating, malnutrition, and malabsorption syndromes, such as Crohn's disease. In addition, many blood pressure medications that cause you to lose water also cause you to lose potassium as you urinate. Kidney problems can cause high levels. If your potassium level is low, you'll be given potassium supplements either by mouth or IV.

Bicarbonate (HCO3) — tells about the carbon dioxide (CO_2) in your body which is influenced by your lungs and kidney functioning. Abnormal levels may suggest that you are losing or retaining fluid, which causes an imbalance in your body's electrolytes. Proper body function requires a balance between the acids and bases. You probably know all about acids and bases if you paid attention in chemistry class!

Blood Urea Nitrogen (BUN) — tells us how your kidneys are functioning. When this level is high, it tells us the waste products, made when your body breaks down protein, aren't being excreted properly or there is an increase in their production. Dehydration and bleeding can raise BUN levels.

Creatinine (Cr) — is another indicator of how well your kidneys are working. When this number is high, we know either body is making more or the kidneys aren't filtering and getting rid of Creatinine properly. Muscle damage and dehydration are often related to an elevated Creatinine level.

Glucose (Glu) — is a type of sugar in your blood. The level fluctuates, depending on what you eat and when and how much energy you're using. When levels are too high, we look for health problems, like diabetes.

Blood Tests for Heart Function

Creatine phosphokinase = Creatine Kinase (CPK or CK) — is an enzyme found in your brain, heart, and skeletal muscles. The level is elevated if there has been injury or stress in these areas. Heart muscle secretes a specific subtype CK called "MB". So if your CK is elevated in your blood and you're having chest pain, they will run the CK-MB to determine if your heart muscle is involved. Remember that your heart is a muscle so the CK is commonly checked when heart involvement is suspected. Repeat isoenzyme CK-MBs may be ordered in 3 hours as levels raise by 3-6 hours after a heart attack. Know that common medications –antibiotics, alcohol and cocaine can effect test results-so be honest about all drugs you are taking.

Troponin (TnI; TnT; cTnI; cTnT) — is an indicator of damaged cardiac muscle. These heart muscle breakdown proteins go into blood stream and are measured in either I form or T form. If the heart has been injured, such as with a heart attack, the level will rise within 6 hours, providing information on the damage. Commonly it is repeated over next 12-16 hours.

C-reactive protein (hs-CRP) - key in identifying heart risk. Likelhood due to inflammation of a heart problems.

Radiology, Imaging Studies

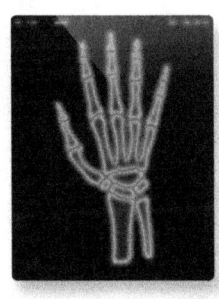

X-Ray and scans (MRI, CT, PET) are valuable imaging tools used to diagnose your problem. Contrary to general opinion, doctors do not have x-ray vision. If you tell the EM doctor you have a pain in your head, he or she may order a test that will help show what is causing the pain. An imaging study may be ordered with or without contrast. The contrast is a solution given by mouth, rectum or IV to help differentiate areas that would otherwise look similar. The contrast may contain iodine so if you are allergic to iodine or shellfish, say so BEFORE the test! There are non-iodinated contrast media. It's also important to let the health care team know if you are or could be pregnant.

A Magnetic Resonance Imager (MRI) is a machine used for diagnostic purposes. Before this test you will be asked if you have any metal in your body, and that includes implanted medical devices and the needle you stepped on 20 years ago that is still there! Metal in an MRI can be lethal so speak up!

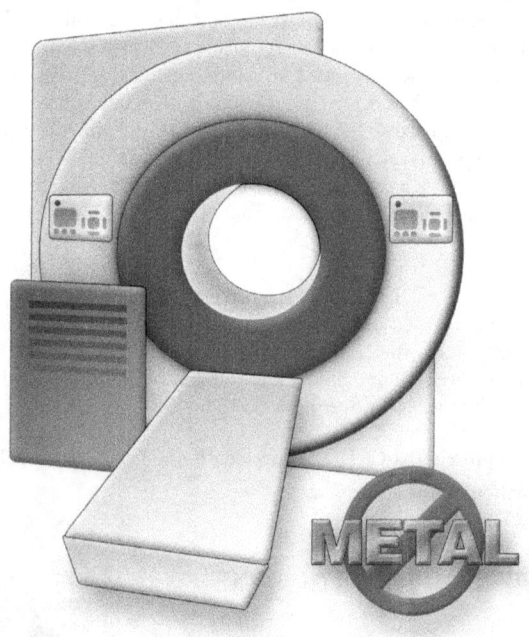

Understand that the results of this test are going to be reviewed and interpreted by a trained radiologist who will share the results with the doctor. And because we're living in the age of technology, this radiologist may not be downstairs in the hospital but on the other side of the world. Preliminary readings are done while you are in the ER; however, you may get a follow-up call if a radiologist makes a different interpretation.

Concern about radiation exposure from medical tests is appropriate. While an imaging study is generally safe, it is not entirely without risk---and not always needed to make a diagnosis. Your doctor will weigh the risks of the study against the benefits it will provide. For example, if a young man presents with the typical signs and symptoms of appendicitis, a CT scan of the abdomen is not necessary to make the diagnosis. On the other hand, a much older person with similar symptoms could have a variety of other diseases and may benefit from a CT of the abdomen.

More is not better, radiation accumulates in our body and can have negative health effects decades later. So question the need for an imaging study if you are not convinced of its merit. Below is a chart that indicates the amount of radiation you are exposed to during certain medical imaging procedures as compared to exposure to natural background radiation.

RADIATION GUIDE

For this procedure:	Your effective radiation dose is:	Comparable to natural background radiation for:
MRI	None	None
Computed Tomography (CT) - Abdomen and Pelvis	10 mSv	3 years
Computed Tomography (CT) - Body	10 mSv	3 years
Radiography - Lower GI Tract	8 mSv	3 years
Radiography - Upper GI Tract	6 mSv	2 years
Radiography - Spine	1.5 mSv	6 months
Radiography - Extremity	0.001 mSv	Less than 1 day
Computed Tomography (CT) - Head	2 mSv	8 months
Computed Tomography (CT) - Spine	6 mSv	2 years
Myelography	4 mSv	16 months
Computed Tomography (CT) - Chest	7 mSv	2 years
Radiographic Chest	0.1 mSv	10 days
Bone Densitometry (DEXA)	0.001 mSv	Less than 1 day
Mammography	0.7 mSv	3 months

Ultrasound (US) imaging, another medical imaging technique used to visualize muscles, tendons, and internal organs, allows recognition of size, structure and any abnormal (pathological) lesions. In an emergency, it can be done at the bedside by a certified EM doctor or ultrasound technician. No radiation is involved. This type of imaging uses sound waves and is safe.

What You Need to Know About Common ER Medical Procedures

Let's be honest, some medical procedures are painful, uncomfortable or embarrassing. But they may be necessary if you want to get well. In this chapter you'll learn about some of the more common ER procedures and get some tips on how to make the best of the experience.

Intravenous (IV) Line Insertion

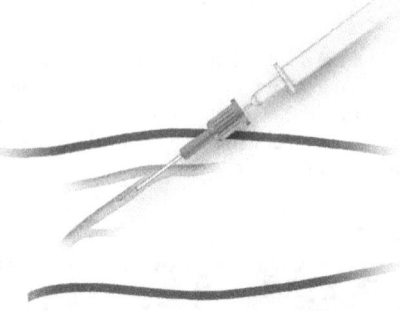

Fluid, blood and medications are given directly into the bloodstream. If required an IV line will be inserted by a nurse or technician. This is a sterile procedure. The nurse must wear gloves and clean the insertion site before placing the introducer needle. A pocket device for illuminating veins can be used in children and hard to find veins. Topical numbing gel can also be used to ease the pain of insertion. Yes, you will feel it when the introducer needle guides the thin walled catheter into the vein but it should be painless afterwards. (No, the needle does NOT stay in your vein. It is used only to break the skin and guide the catheter into the vein.) After the needle is removed the catheter and connection will be securely taped and labeled with the date and time of insertion.

Sometimes it takes multiple attempts to access a vein because of the texture of your veins or because you're dehydrated. (You learned about this earlier when we talked about blood draws.) The nurse should make only two attempts before asking someone else to try. If you have discomfort from the IV once it is in, speak up! It might not be properly positioned.

If, after it is inserted and fluids are running, you notice oozing around the tape or increased swelling, redness or pain at the site, let the nurse know right away. The IV may have become dislodged from the vein, resulting in leakage into the surrounding tissues. When this is the case, the IV has to be taken out and a new one inserted, always in a different location. If your skin is swollen and red, ask for warm compress.

You can help to prevent this from happening by keeping your hand away from the IV site. Don't pull or play with the tubing. Separated tubing connections causes oozing and leakage. If the IV machine beeps, don't touch it. Let your nurse know.

You aren't trained or authorized to operate the machine and could give yourself too much medication if you start playing with the settings.

An IV can be a 'hep lock' (heparin lock) that is access is ready but no tubing/flow is present. Medication into your vein can be given through a 'hep lock' IV via a syringe push. A push of medication followed by a flush solution to move medication and keep the vein from clotting. An IV must be removed before you can leave the hospital. Don't leave with one in your arm and please don't take it out yourself; it is not like in the movies! Any improper attempt at removal may result in bleeding and infection. Ask your nurse to remove it.

Monitoring Your Heart

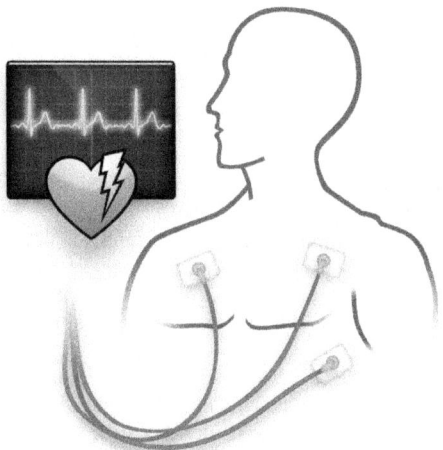

If you're in the ER because of chest pain, or you have a cardiac history, you will have an Electrocardiogram (ECG, also called EKG) done and after may remain hooked up to a cardiac monitor. An ECG does not hurt but requires you to lie still and silent during the test. You will be attached to a recording machine by several sticky pasties placed across the chest and on your limbs or sides. ECG machines record the electrical activity of your heart as lines (wave forms) on a small strip of graph paper. The computer records several beats simultaneously, as viewed from 12 or 16 sides of the heart. Most ECG machines are capable of interpreting the tracing as it prints the paper copy. The 'machine' interpretation is not to take the place of a doctor's interpretation.

This brings up an important point: Any test that is performed is looked at by a doctor and interpreted in light of your complaint and physical examination. Remember, you are being treated not the test results.

Nasogastric (NG) Tube Insertion

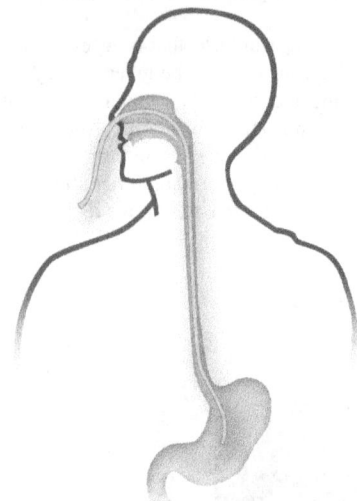

A quick way to get things in or out of the stomach is to insert a NG tube. It is used to relieve pressure caused by fluid behind an obstruction or to remove blood or stomach acid. ER staff will estimate the distance from your nostril to your stomach first. A soft, clear tube is placed through one nostril and travels down your throat and into your stomach. Yes, you are awake for this! Yes, it is uncomfortable. Here are a few things that might make the process less distressing:

- Speak up if you have had a broken nose, deviated septum or sinus surgery. This information will help determine which nostril should be used. It is best to use an unobstructed nostril.

- A clear jelly anesthetic is usually placed in the nostril or around the tube tip. If not request it.

- Insist, if not already done, that the tube be placed in ice water first. This stiffens the tube and makes it glide more easily. The tip of the tube should be well lubricated.

- Stay calm. Yes, it is uncomfortable but the benefits will outweigh the discomfort. Trust me on this one.

- Bend your neck into your chest as you sip on ice water best through a straw, when instructed. The tube will pass easier if you swallow when instructed.

- Once inserted, the nurse must verify the tube's placement in your stomach before putting anything in the tube. A medical staff member should listen for a rush of air as air is injected into the tube and/or a chest x-ray should be taken to verify placement.

- GI Cocktail – Don't get too excited when you hear you're going to get a cocktail with your new NG tube! There's no such thing as happy hour in the ER. Most commonly given by mouth for chest pain or pain in the upper abdomen, the gastrointestinal (GI) cocktail is a therapeutic oral mix of liquid preparations to help in the diagnosis and treatment of GI problems.

Breathing Aids

Your care may include oxygen administration. Oxygen is administered through nasal prongs or a facemask. It will be adjusted according to your oxygenation level. Your oxygenation level is measured by attaching a monitoring device to your finger. For infants, the device is attached to the baby's toes. The amount of oxygen you receive is guided by the result on a monitor or blood test. Unlike Mae West, more is not always better.

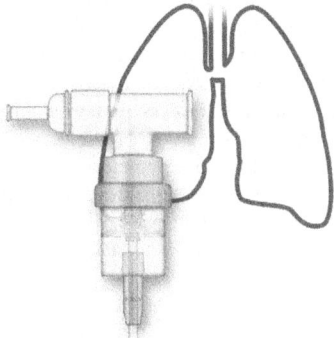

If you require a breathing treatment to help you breathe better, the medication will be given through a jet nebulizer and administered by a respiratory technician or nurse who will stay by your side throughout the treatment. As you breathe, the medication will be forced into your lungs through a connection to a compressed air or oxygen source. If, during treatment, you experience a sensation out of the ordinary speak up. Before and after the treatment your peak expiratory flow rate (PEFR) will be measured with a meter. It is best to conduct this measurement while standing, if your condition permits. You'll be asked to exhale rapidly and forcefully with lips sealed around the meter's mouthpiece. This allows your EM doctor to determine if there has been measurable improvement in your breathing. Age and height are factors important in determining normal PEFR.

Closing a Wound

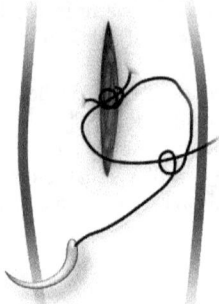

If you come in with a cut (that's what we call a wound or laceration) that needs to be closed, here's what to expect: first, the wound will be cleaned thoroughly before it is closed in order to prevent infection. The EM doctor and nurse will be following sterile procedure, which includes wearing sterile gloves, to avoid getting any bacteria into the wound. So please, don't touch anything.

Whether or not staples, thread (suture material) or glue is used depends on the size and location of the wound. If sutures are used, you'll be interested to know that thread size is a consideration. Different synthetic threads are assigned a number that refers to tensile strength; the higher the number the finer the thread. Suture material can be made of silk or synthetic material connected to curve needles of varying sizes. For instance, fine thread like "6-0" is often used on the face. Ask your doctor what size thread she's using and you'll get her attention. A trained 'suture technician' may be told by the EM doctor to clean and 'close' your laceration. Certain very large lacerations will need to be repaired in the operating room and may require referral to general surgeon or a plastic surgeon. Complicated facial lacerations might need to be evaluated by a plastic surgeon.

Different parts of the body heal at different rates, for example sutures in the face normally come out in three to five days. Dissolving sutures (absorbable) are used to close lower layers that are under tension. They can take a month to absorb. On the leg, which is further away from the heart skin take longer to heal so sutures may be left in for weeks. If sutures are over a joint, the joint will be immobilized to help healing and reduce scaring. Do not remove your own sutures. If you notice any swelling, drainage, redness or heat, especially after 48 hours, call your doctor.

Cast and Splint

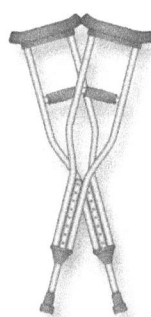

A fractured bone is a broken bone is a cracked bone. It may be displaced and need to be put back into alignment. Don't worry; you'll be given IV sedation for this. This is called a 'reduction'. Some fractures cause the bone to penetrate the skin. This is an orthopedic emergency, requiring an urgent orthopedic consultation and a visit to the OR. Some fractures can be splinted and will heal on their own. Some fractures require casts or an 'ortho glass' splint. Other fractures, like rib fractures, require no treatment except pain control.

If you did not break a bone you may have sustained a sprain, which is a torn ligament fibers, causing swelling pain and inability of the limb to function normally. Sprains are graded by the resulting loss of joint support. These are treated according to the degree with elastic wrap, splint, cast or even surgery for a complete ligament tear! If your ankle or knee is sprained you will likely be given crutches. Sprains can take weeks to heal. You will be measured for and taught how to use your crutches. Pay attention---you do not want another injury!

It is your responsibility to speak up if a treatment is causing pain. It's also important to follow instructions regarding splints, slings, crutches, or casts. Failure to follow instructions could delay healing. Let a doctor know if you notice numbness or significant increase in pain without injury. Be aware that discomfort from a fracture can last four to eight weeks as the bone heals.

A fracture happens in a second but takes months to heal. The good news is that it gets better with time, rather than worse. Your doctor, to get you back to your old self, may prescribe special exercises and rehabilitation.

Nerve Block

This refers to an injection of medication in/about a nerve that connects with the painful area. Used for the purpose of giving anesthetic medication, it is commonly done for rib fractures. Blocks are also used to anesthetize an area for painless skin repair (suturing).

Joint Tap

Trauma, disease and infection can cause a bone joint to swell from fluid collection. After an x-ray and for further testing or pain relief, a 'tap' may be done. This involves using a needled syringe to enter the joint space and remove fluid or blood for possible testing. The EM doctor does this procedure. Yes the area is numbed first. In addition, medications may be injected to help treat the condition.

Foley Catheter Insertion

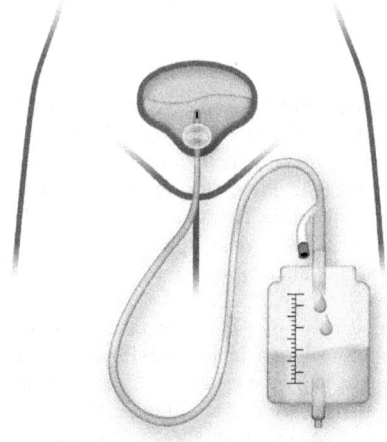

When the nurse comes in and says, "we're going to put in a Foley" here's what's going to happen. A Foley is a device designed to continuously drain your bladder of urine. Once inserted, you won't have to get out of bed to void (urinate). The urine will drain on its own into a collection bag. There are many benefits to having one, including not waiting for a TV commercial to go to the bathroom. If you're immobilized by your injury or illness, you won't have to be rolled on and off bedpans. In addition, your urine output is an indicator of your fluid balance so it is important for the medical staff to have an accurate picture of your output. Yes, insertion is uncomfortable.

You're going to have to lie flat on your back for this procedure. Women will be asked to bend their knees and spread their legs. This is a sterile procedure. Your genital area will be cleaned carefully before the sterile tube is inserted. If you are allergic to iodine or shellfish, speak up. Chances are the cleanser commonly used is iodine based. After cleansing, the lubricated tip of the tube will be inserted to the point when urine starts to flow. Men with prostate swelling may experience significant discomfort as the tube enters and is tunneled to the bladder. Once the tip is in your bladder, urine flows as an indicator it is in the right spot.

Here's what a Foley looks like and how it stays put. The tip of the tubing has an inflatable balloon that anchors in the bladder. The balloon is filled with about a tablespoon of sterile water once inserted to hold it in place. The solution is removed when it is time to take out the Foley, deflating the balloon and allowing the tube to slide out easily. So please, don't tug on the tubing or try to take it out on your own. It will hurt and could injure you.

The catheter tubing is anchored against your thigh to stabilize it. Notice where the drainage bag is. The urine collected will be emptied and measured so leave it alone!

Straight Catheterization

If a clean urine sample is needed, the same procedure for inserting a Foley is followed except no bag is necessary and the catheter is removed after the specimen is collected. This procedure is often done on children when a clean urine specimen is necessary for testing.

Incision & Drainage "I & D"

When a boil turns into an abscess (large collection of pus) it might need to be opened, drained, cleaned and then packed in order for it to heal. This might be done by the EM doctor or by a surgeon in the OR. This is a painful procedure so it is often done in the OR.

CHAPTER 5
Medical Dynamics

Your Role As A Patient

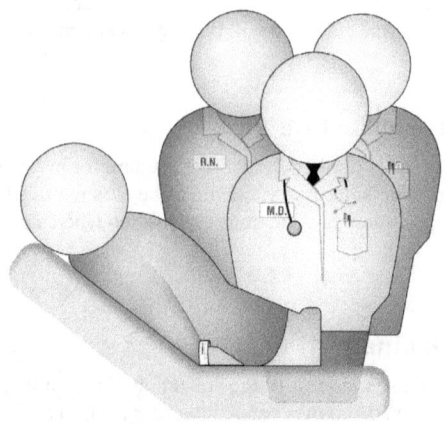

By now, you should have a good picture of what an ER visit will be like. Here's what you can do to help ensure you get the best care possible:

- Present your problem and medical history clearly and succinctly. Refer to your notes and Health History Sheet (Medical History / Medication List), Pocket Med Card and be honest.

- Get to know the staff. Call them by name. If you're not sure who they are or what their job is, ask.

- If you don't understand something, or a person speaks too fast, ask them to repeat what was said. If there's a language barrier, request a translator.

- If you don't understand why you're getting a specific test or medication, ask for clarification. There's always a chance they've got the wrong person.

- Provide your name and date of birth when asked (and when not asked), to be sure they have the right patient for the right test or medication.

- Make your needs known. If you're cold, ask for a blanket. If you're in pain, ask if you can have pain meds.

- Stay put. Don't leave your assigned area.

- Prevent falls by allowing staff to help you get on stretcher, wheelchair, or assist you to the bathroom. Falls are common in the ER because people are weaker than they think. Ask for help.

- Follow instructions.

- Don't eat or drink unless allowed.

- Don't touch equipment. If the IV machine beeps, notify your nurse. Don't try to change settings even though you've seen the nurse do it a dozen times.

- Don't empty your urinal or emesis basin. The nurse may need to measure, test and/or assess the contents.

- Don't try to help other patients. They're not your responsibility and you could do more harm than good. Help them by calling the nurse.

- Appoint one family member as liaison in order to limit the number of visitors and phone calls. Choose someone who is a good listener and will stay calm and help the medical staff. This person should be familiar with your health history and medications, whenever possible.

- Give valuables to family member or ask nurse to get hospital security to lock them up.

Your Role As Family / Friend

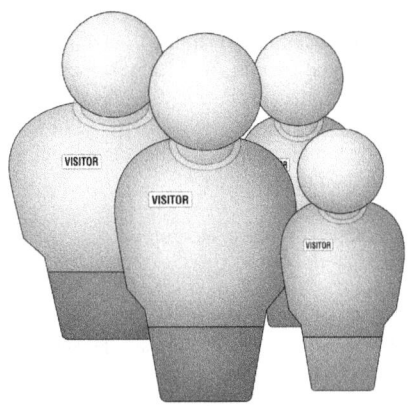

If a friend or family member is taken to the ER, here's what you can do to help.

- Appoint one person to serve as liaison between hospital staff and family to minimize the number of phone calls and conversations with staff. Staff time will be wasted repeating information.

- Stay calm. Don't make a scene.

- Describe any pre-hospital changes seen in the patient that the patient might not have mentioned.

- Notify the nurse if you notice a change in the patient, such as a change in mental status, sweating, or increased weakness.

- Don't give the patient anything to eat or drink unless permitted by the nurse.

- Don't touch equipment. If a machine starts to beep don't try to stop it. Notify the nurse. Never touch equipment settings even if you've seen the nurse reset the machine and think you can do it.

- Use your cell phone in designated areas. This will help to ensure your friend's privacy, as well as keeping the noise level down in the treatment area.

- Don't plug in any computers, CDs or other electronic devices into hospital electrical outlets. And don't use these devices on battery without checking with the nurse first. There are reports of personal electronic devices interfering with hospital equipment. Some electronic devices have also been known to threaten implantable rhythm devices, such as pacemakers and defibrillators.

- Limit and control number of visitors. Ill and immune compromised family members and friends should stay home and check in by phone instead.

- Prevent falls by not allowing the patient to get out of bed without first checking with the nurse.

- Respect the patient's privacy and don't repeat what you hear without the patient's agreement.

- Stay healthy. Wash your hands often. Use hand sanitizer. Get some rest and eat well-balanced meals. Having an ill or injured family member or friend can be stressful on you, as well.

- Advocate for your patient by reminding healthcare workers to wash their hands and wear gloves.

- Don't try to help other patients. Notify the nurse or other healthcare provider.

- Leave children at home, if possible. If that's not possible, clean their hands and toys often. Don't let them crawl around on the hospital floor.

- Stay in one spot so staff can find you.

- Respect other people's privacy. If you see someone in the ER that you know, or hear something about someone, don't share that information. Treat other people's privacy with respect.

- Don't socialize. You're in the ER, not the shopping mall. This is not the time or place to socialize.

- Don't empty patient's urinal or emesis basin. Vomit or urine may need to be measured or assessed.

- Use restrooms for visitors, not the ones in patient areas.

Complaints

Lighten up! Don't go into the ER with an attitude that it is going to go badly. Understand that there are days and times when challenges are overwhelming to all parties concerned. However, if your ER visit isn't going smoothly, here's what you do. Get your notes together and explain your concern to your nurse. If your nurse can't resolve the issue, or the nurse is the issue, start going up the chain of command. Every hospital has a chain of command and a grievance process for handling complaints. Typically, the levels go something like this while you're in the ER:

1. Nurse
2. Charge Nurse
3. Nursing Supervisor
4. Patient Advocate or Patient Relations
5. ER Administrator

Don't lose your focus! Other ill and injured people in the ER need attention, too. Present yourself and your complaint in a manner that will promote cooperation.

Once you leave the ER, you can also file a formal complaint with the hospital or with the state public health department or medical board. Both have formal grievance processes regarding service and treatment in a medical facility.

In addition, if your hospital is accredited by the Joint Commission (over 20,000 health care organizations), you can voice your complaints through this organization by: completing on line form, by writing: Office of Quality & Patient Safety, The Joint Commission, One Renaissance Boulevard, Oakbrook Terrace, IL 60181 or by calling 1-800-994-6610.

CHAPTER 6

Leaving The ER

Disposition – (Leaving the ER)

Once your workup is complete, discussed with you and a care plan made, it is time to leave the ER. Where you go depends on what's wrong with you. You may be admitted, held for observation, transferred to another facility, or sent home. Your discharge from the ER, like your admission, takes time. It's not like a hotel where you can check out any time you wish. Your EM doctor must write a discharge order before you go anywhere. If you decide to leave before receiving discharge instructions, this is considered leaving Against Medical Advice (AMA), you may not only risk your life but your insurance may not pay for your care. Think about this carefully and weigh your options before you act.

Let's review each discharge option and discuss what to expect.

Admission To The Hospital

Please understand that the hospital has to find the appropriate bed for you and this may take time. Again, this is not a hotel! There are only so many beds for a specific type of medical problem; you can't take a 'med/surg' bed if you need to go to the Intensive Care Unit (ICU). Most in-hospital rooms are semi-private. Private rooms are usually assigned to persons who require isolation or have special needs, such as hospice care. If you want a private room, and there's no medical reason for you to have one, you may be expected to pay the additional fees out of your own pocket. Depending on the occupancy rate (census) in the hospital, you may have to wait until someone is discharged and the room is cleaned before moving to your room. In some situations, this can take many hours.

In the meantime, documentation of your care in the ER, whether electronic or handwritten, has to be completed and a report sent to your next destination. You should give your valuables to your family member or to hospital security for safekeeping. Personal items, like a toothbrush, gown and slippers will be provided by the hospital. While you're waiting, you are still a patient in the ER and it is important that you continue to make sure your needs are met. A nurse is assigned to you and responsible for your care.

Once admitted to the hospital, it's not likely that your personal doctor or the EM doctor will be taking care of you. Instead, you will be under the care of the Hospitalists. These doctors are usually in the hospital 24/7 and will likely come to the ER to exam and continue or start your needed care.

In teaching hospitals you will be admitted to a "service". Each medical specialty has a "service" with Residents and an Attending physician taking admissions from the ER. So you probably won't see your personal care physician (PCP) in the hospital, but it is a good idea to let him or her know you have been admitted and why. The Resident of the 'service' or the Hospitalist can always call your PCP if they have any concerns or questions. The good news is that you'll go back to your PCP once discharged.

Observation

A third of US hospitals already have observation units where you can be admitted for a stay of less than 24 hours. If you have been in the ER for 12 hours and admission is not warranted but you require close monitoring, intense treatment, you can go to the observation unit. Insurance pays for this special unit but not for 'observation status' so ask. Remember to learn the specifics of your health insurance coverage long in advance. Providers actually prefer this step for certain diagnoses/conditions such as: Back pain, Transfusion, Dehydration, Asthma. This allows time for further evaluation and treatment of conditions likely to improve within 24 hours. During this time, care that would be difficult to give at home is provided by a dedicated team following specific protocols. Again, you'll be transferred to the observation unit when a bed is available. 'Admitted for Observation' is not the same as admitted to the hospital, this becomes important for health insurance reasons, so ask.

Transfer

Whether due to need for specialized care, insurance reasons or personal choice arrangements for a transfer to another facility can take time. You may be admitted until the arrangements are complete. In addition to arranging for your admission to the other facility, the hospital has to coordinate your transportation and seek authorization. Important is that the receiving facility has to accept you in transfer.

Discharge To Home

If you're going home, the EM doctor has to write your discharge order and follow-up instructions. If you do not have a personal physician, one will be assigned to you. Prescriptions for medications related to your complaint will be provided. If it is the middle of the night, a few doses of your meds may be given to tide you over until you can get your prescription(s) filled. It's not the ER's responsibility to reorder your cholesterol medication or birth control pills so please don't ask. The nurse will review the paperwork with you and complete the discharge documents. Remember, both the nurse and the EM doctor are taking care of other patients and prioritizing who needs them first. You've been cared for so it may take a while for the paperwork to be completed.

After the discharge instructions and follow-up recommendations are carefully explained you will be asked to sign them, verifying that you received the instructions and that you understand them. A copy of the document you sign goes into your medical record so be sure you are clear on what you must do. Your signature means that you understand. You'll receive a copy of your discharge instructions to take with you. If, after you leave, it is determined that test result information requires further action, you will be notified.

Always remember it is your responsibility to:

- Ask questions. While you're waiting to be discharged, take out your pen and paper and make a list of questions you want answered before you leave the ER.

- Review the discharge instructions and make sure you understand what you have to do.

- Make sure you understand any new medicine prescriptions.

  o *What is the medicine for? What time should I take it? How much should I take? Should I take it with food? Are there any side effects? What should I do if I miss a dose? Can I take it with my other medications? Are there any food, drink, or activities I should avoid while on this medication? How long should I take it?*

- Request that a record of your visit be sent to your primary care physician. For some hospitals, it will be electronically sent, others you may have to send a request to their medical records department. You also can do this after you're discharged.

- Return if your symptoms don't resolve. If you have followed the instructions and do not continue to improve or your condition worsens, follow up with your own doctor or return to the ER. You won't be the first person who has returned to the ER and you won't be the last. If you feel you need emergency assistance, don't hesitate to call 911/EMS.

- Provide feedback on your visit to the ER when asked. Feedback is used to help improve conditions. Don't just focus on the negative aspects give constructive criticism. Praise staff when appropriate.

- Discard your bracelet once at home. Eliminate the opportunity for someone else to use your health information.

- Follow up with appointments, lab work or other diagnostic studies. If your follow-up appointment is scheduled for the next day make sure you get a copy of any test results if the doctor you are assigned won't have access to them. It's important to bring any documents given to you in the ER to your follow-up appointments.

CHAPTER 7
Deciphering Medical Jargon

Like any other area of work, the ER has its own language, often comprised of abbreviations and acronyms used to save time and space — something like texting. For example, "SOB" in the medical world stands for "short of breath" not, well you know. As part of your inside view of the ER, I've put together a list of common lingo you might hear around the ER.

ABG (Arterial Blood Gas) - a blood test to measure your exact blood oxygen level and other critical values

ALS (Advanced Life Support) - resuscitation using drugs and connection to machine(s)

AMA (Against Medical Advice) - leaving the hospital against the advice of your doctor and without a discharge order

Angina Pectoris - chest pain from heart disease

AOB (Alcohol on Breath)

ARRA (American Recovery and Reinvestment Act of 2009) – aspects adresse the health care delivery system and payements

Block - refers to injecting a nerve to stop it from transmitting impulses, the most common of which is pain

BP - blood pressure reading

CABG (Coronary Artery Bypass Graft) - An operation (open heart surgery) in which a piece of vein or artery is used as a graft to bypass a blockage in a coronary artery; performed to prevent myocardial infarction and relieve angina pectoris

CAD (Coronary Artery Disease) - Atherosclerosis (hardening) of the arteries to the heart

CATH (catheterization) - passing a catheter into arteries to see if there is narrowing, commonly used to study the heart and place stents

CHF (Congestive Heart Failure) - condition where the heart is unable to pump efficiently, resulting in fluid retention in the tissues and shortness of breath

Cocktail- multiple medications given together to have an improved effect

CODE - refers to resuscitation attempts to restore breathing and circulation

COPD (Chronic Obstructive Pulmonary Disease) – emphysema

CT - or "CAT", refers to an imaging study that looks inside the body as cross-sectional images

CVA (Cerebral Vascular Accident) - a blockage or rupture of a blood vessel in or around your brain, also referred to as "stroke"

DNAR (Do Not Attempt Resuscitation) or DNR (Do Not Resuscitate)

DOA (Dead on Arrival) used when no resuscitative effort is made due to state of the body

ECG or EKG (electrocardiogram) - a test that measures and shows the electrical activity of the heart muscle

EME bag – disposable bag to vomit (emesis) into

EMR or EHR electronic health or medical record

EMS (Emergency Medical Services) - collectively refers to ambulance response system, including paramedics and EMTs

ETOH - refers to alcohol use or intoxication

FOS (Full of Stool) - arrived at as a finding when exam or X-ray reveals presence of a large amount of stool in colon

Hook up - attach equipment devices to patient to monitor blood pressure, oxygen and heart rhythm

ICD (Implantable Cardioverter Defibrillator) - a device under the skin with a wire in the heart that can sense and deliver electrical energy as needed to keep the heart in normal rhythm

ICE (in case of emergency) – person who knows your medical history

ICU (Intensive Care Unit) - area in the hospital for critical patients requiring very close monitoring

I&D (incision & drainage) - procedure to open and clean a collection of pus

IM (intramuscular) - refers to an injection given into the muscle

IV (intravenous,) - a way to give you medication, fluid or blood through your vein

KVO (Keep Vein Open) - refers to a flow rate to 'run' IV fluids into your vein, usually a very slow rate

MI (Myocardial Infarction) - heart attack, meaning the heart muscle is dying

MRI (Magnetic Resonance Imaging) - using a magnetic scanning device to provide a detailed view of a particular area inside the body

MVA (motor vehicle accident)

NG Tube (Nasogastric Tube) - tube inserted through your nose into your stomach

NPO (nothing by mouth) - means you can't eat or drink anything

O2 (oxygen)

OD (Oculus Dexter) - right eye

OS (Oculus Sinister) - left eye

OU (Oculi Unitio) - both eyes

PA (Physician Assistant)

PATCH - EMS personnel communicating with the hospital while en route

PET scan (Positron Emission Tomography) - shows how organs and tissues are functioning, i.e. blood flow, oxygen use, and sugar (glucose) metabolism

PCP (Personal Care Physician)

PFA (Patient Financial Advisor) - healthcare facility personnel that work on payment issues with you.

PO - by mouth

Push - refers to injecting a medication rapidly into a vein

ROM (Range of Motion) - refers to joint movement in degrees

RN (Registered Nurse)

RN-P (Registered Nurse Practitioner) or APRN (Advanced Practice Registered Nurse)

SCAN - imaging studies, most commonly an MRI, CT or PET

SOB - short of breath

SQ (subcutaneous) - injection given just under the skin

SVN (small volume nebulizer) - a 'machine' that turns liquid medication into an aerosol so the medication can be inhaled and delivered to your lungs; sometimes called a "breathing treatment" or "neb treatment"

Strip - an ECG tracing of your heart activity off a monitor

T-boned - a motor vehicle collision impacting the side of one of the vehicles

TIA (Transient Ischemic Attack) - temporary loss of speech or limb function, often referred to as a "mini stroke" that may herald a major stroke

UA (Urine Analysis) - a lab test to exam urine for infection or chemical abnormalities

UDS (Ultrasound Doppler Sonogram) - a study that uses differences in sound wave transmission to visualize internal structures